**Prentice-Hall Series
in the Philosophy of Medicine**

Samuel Gorovitz,
Series Editor

Man,

and

The Ethics

Samuel Gorovitz
Series Editor

Prentice-Hall, Inc., Englewood Cliffs 07632

Mind, Morality

of Behavior Control

RUTH MACKLIN

Department of Community Health
Albert Einstein College of Medicine

P 70

174.2
M15m

Library of Congress Cataloging in Publication Data

MACKLIN, RUTH
  Man, mind, and morality.
  (Prentice-Hall series in the philosophy of
medicine)
    Bibliography:
    Includes index.
    1. Psychiatric ethics. 2. Psychotherapy ethics.
  3. Control (Psychology.) I. Title. II. Title:
  Behavior control. III. Series.
  RC455.2.E8M32   174'.2   81-4339
  ISBN 0-13-551127-5   AACR2

JM

Printed in the United States of America

10   9   8   7   6   5   4   3   2   1

PRENTICE-HALL INTERNATIONAL, INC., *London*
PRENTICE-HALL OF AUSTRALIA PTY. LIMITED, *Sydney*
PRENTICE-HALL OF CANADA, LTD., *Toronto*
PRENTICE-HALL OF INDIA PRIVATE LIMITED, *New Delhi*
PRENTICE-HALL OF JAPAN, INC., *Tokyo*
PRENTICE-HALL OF SOUTHEAST ASIA PTE. LTD., *Singapore*
WHITEHALL BOOKS LIMITED, WELLINGTON, *New Zealand*

**To my mother
and the memory of my father**

Contents

Freedom versus Coercion *41*

Therapy and Social Control *59*

Institutions and Alternatives *79*

Behavior Control in a Free Society: Treatment and Research *101*

Preface
to the Series

It is a commonplace observation that there have been dramatic increases both in public and professional concern with questions of bioethics and in the role of philosophers in addressing those questions. Medical ethics is a well established area of inquiry; not only does it include journals, widespread courses, professional specialists, and the other features of established fields, but philosophers now participate regularly in the deliberations of public agencies at both state and federal levels. Nonetheless, there is considerably more to the philosophy of medicine than medical ethics, and even within the area of medical ethics, there are many issues that have not been adequately explored.

The Prentice-Hall Series in the Philosophy of Medicine has been established in large measure in response to these two points. Some volumes in the series will explore philosophical aspects of medicine that are not primarily questions of ethics. They thereby contribute both to the subject matter of the philosophy of medicine and to an expanding appreciation of the breadth and diversity of the philosophy of medicine. Other volumes in the series will illuminate areas of ethical concern which, despite the recent prominence of medical ethics, have been inadequately considered.

Each volume is written by a philosopher, although none is written primarily for philosophers. Rather, the volumes are designed to bring the issues before an intelligent general readership, and they therefore presuppose no specific background in either the philosophical literature or the literature of the specific areas of medical practice or health policy on which they focus.

The problems considered in this series are of widespread public importance. We suffer from no delusions that philosophers hold the solutions; we do, however, share the conviction that these problems cannot be adequately addressed without an informed appreciation of their philosophical dimensions. We must always reach beyond philosophy in addressing problems in the world, but we should be wary of reaching without it. The volumes in this series are thus addressed to all those concerned with the practices and policies relating to medicine and health, and committed to considering such policies in a reflective and rational way.

SAMUEL GOROVITZ

Acknowledgments

Past work of the Behavior Control Research Group of the Hastings Center, Institute of Society, Ethics and the Life Sciences, was an invaluable resource to me in shaping the contents of this book. My colleague, Willard Gaylin, contributed many ideas to that work, and some of those have, no doubt, found their way into my thinking. He and I have not always agreed on precise formulations or substantive moral views, but I am indebted to him for launching my thoughts on a number of these topics. I want to thank Sam Gorovitz and Peggy Battin, who read and commented on earlier versions of the manuscript. And I am grateful to all those who assisted in research, typing, and other tasks: Meryl Macklin, Bonnie Baya, Eva Mannheimer, Mary Gualandi, Carola Mone, Shelley Macklin, and David Wolk. I would also like to thank Milton F. Shore, Mental Health Study Center, National Institute of Mental Health, Adelphi, Maryland, who reviewed the manuscript and made many helpful comments.

This work was supported in part by the National Science Foundation, grant number OSS77-17072, in a joint award with the National Endowment for the Humanities.

CHAPTER 1

Behavior Control
and Morality

Almost all our major problems involve human behavior, and they cannot be solved by physical and biological technology alone. What is needed is a technology of behavior, but we have been slow to develop the science from which such a technology might be drawn.... It will not solve our problems, however, until it replaces traditional prescientific views, and these are strongly entrenched. Freedom and dignity illustrate the traditional theory, and they are essential to practices in which a person is held responsible for his conduct and given credit for his achievements. A scientific analysis shifts both the responsibility and the achievement to the environment. It also raises questions concerning "values." Who will use a technology and to what ends? Until these issues are resolved, a technology of behavior will continue to be rejected, and with it possibly the only way to solve our problems.

B. F. Skinner
Beyond Freedom and Dignity

That which constitutes the condition under which alone anything can be an end in itself, this has not merely a relative worth, *i.e.,* value, but an intrinsic worth, that is *dignity.... Autonomy* then is the basis of the dignity of human and of every rational nature.... What else then can freedom of the will be but autonomy, that is the property of the will to be a law to itself?... Now the idea of freedom is inseparably connected with the conception of *autonomy,* and this again with the universal principle of morality which is ideally the foundation of all actions of *rational* beings, just as the law of nature is of all phenomena.

Immanuel Kant
Fundamental Principles of the Metaphysics of Morals

The Issues

A murderer sentenced to life imprisonment is subjected to a form of behavior control: His liberty to move freely about and thus to act in certain undesirable ways is taken away. Parents who give their children a dollar for every A on their report cards are trying to shape behavior by the method psychologists call "positive reinforcement": They reward behavior they approve of with something desirable in the hope that the "good" behavior will be repeated. The behavior of a patient about to enter the operating room is controlled by a shot of morphine: This is designed to calm the patient—emotionally as well as physically—before surgery. Some people prone to violent outbursts resulting from an abnormal brain condition known as "temporal lobe epilepsy" even seek to control their own behavior: they choose to have extremely delicate brain surgery that helps prevent these outbursts.

The term "behavior control" has an ominous ring to it. Why is this? For one thing, it conjures up a medieval image of the rack or thumbscrew—modes of human torture once used widely but repugnant to modern moral sentiments. Whether it is used as punishment for past acts or as a means of coercion, as in getting suspects to reveal information, torture as a form of behavior control is ruled out on moral grounds. In addition, the term "behavior control" raises visions of sinister scientists with powerful devices designed to change people's behavior and even to alter their whole personalities. But we need not turn to science fiction to find examples of psychotechnology developed and used foı the express purpose of controlling people's behavior. In recent years the advances have been striking in both psychological theory and medical technology, making it possible to change a person's mood, behavior, thought, and emotion. These techniques are offered and promoted under the guise of therapy or rehabilitation. Brain surgeons possess skill and know-how enabling them to perform refined and delicate acts of psychosurgery. Strides in psychopharmacology make it possible to deaden, pep up, or calm people whose levels of anxiety or daily mood swings are not desirable to them or to other people. These powerful new therapeutic technologies have brought with them special ethical and legal dilemmas never before experienced.

But there are also conceptual questions. Should every attempt to influence another person's thoughts, feelings, or actions be considered an act of behavior control? Or does the term "behavior control" refer only to practices aimed at eliminating "bad" behavior, rather than to a broader range of acts that include encouraging excellence or improvement? These are conceptual questions about the meaning and scope of the term "behavior control." There is no clear, single meaning of this concept, although certain uses may be preferable for certain purposes.

In this book I employ the notion of behavior control in its broadest sense, to include everything from weak forms of emotional or intellectual influence and subtle efforts to shape ideas, to various modes of psychotherapy, to invasive procedures that alter the brain or the chemical workings of the body. What this usage lacks in precision, it gains in comprehensiveness and easy reference to a variety of ways of altering people's psychological dispositions. This usage makes it possible to mark off weaker and stronger modes of influence or control. It also suggests the need to distinguish among the following: efforts aimed at altering thought patterns; attempts to change mood or feelings; and methods that seek to change behavior directly, bypassing the rational processes. Though the broad use of "behavior control'' adopted here may seem arbitrary to some, it is one of several standard ways of referring to the wide range of topics the term may denote.

Although in earlier eras people did not have the scientific knowledge and technological refinements that abound today, they have always practiced methods of behavior control in one form or another. Behavior can be molded and personality shaped by a variety of activities: Nurturing during infancy, educating in childhood and adolescence, and special modes of training such as those used in the military or athletics are only a few common examples. The very existence of methods for controlling behavior is a universal fact of life in all structured societies. But whatever form these methods actually take in any culture, it is likely that ethical issues will lurk somewhere about.

As used here, the terms ''morality'' and ''ethics'' refer to a set of normative principles, or accepted practices, whose purpose is to guide the conduct of people toward one another. The fact that different cultures exhibit a wide variety of moral codes and practices raises the perennial problem of ethical relativism, . . . the question of whether it is sound for acts or practices to be morally right in one society, yet wrong in another. Still, because every culture faces *some* ethical choices, the rules that govern behavior and the penalties for violating those rules must have some connection with a system of ethics. This book will confine its examination of behavior control to practices, norms, and dilemmas in contemporary Western society.

New Problems Introduced by Technology

Ethical issues arising out of efforts aimed at controlling behavior have always been with us. But now the choices made possible by at least some of the new technologies raise moral concerns requiring decision and action on the part of judges, of legislatures, of those who run institutions—schools, hospitals, prisons—where behavior-control technologies are already in use or proposed; and, last but not least, of individuals of the general population themselves.

What are these ethical issues and how are moral problems involving behavior control to be resolved? One question gets directly to the heart of the matter: Who may do what to whom, and with what justification? The following considerations, at least, are morally relevant to answering this question.

—The type or nature of technological manipulation, or intervention: Does it have consequences that are reversible (as is believed to be the case for most, but not all, drugs used for therapy)? Is it irreversible, as is oft noted with horror about even the most refined techniques of psychosurgery? Is the technique highly invasive, such as cutting open the head or implanting electrodes in the brain? And if so, what bearing does this have?

—What the behavior-control technique aims at changing: Compare the difference between removing small, yet unwanted behavior patterns such as fingernail biting or more important types of behavior such as smoking, on the one hand; and on the other, wholesale personality changes, including such ideological transformations as ''brainwashing,'' and dramatic religious conversions, as well as their alleged ''cure''—deprogramming.

—The urgency of producing change: What makes the need for change urgent? One reason might be the severity of the behavior—the likelihood of causing social harm or some form of permanent damage to the self, unless there is behavior change.

—The purpose for which behavior change is sought, as well as the nature of the population involved: Is the change aimed at rehabilitating criminal offenders? "Curing" the mentally ill? Making the retarded more self-reliant and independent? Getting rid of unwanted habits or undesirable traits? Enhancing performance or increasing levels of skill? It is important to recall that techniques used to control behavior can be used to promote excellence and foster improvement in people, as well as to change or eliminate undesirable traits or patterns of actions.

—The feasibility of gaining the informed consent of the person whose behavior is being altered: Is truly informed consent ever possible? Can such consent ever or usually be given voluntarily by institutionalized persons? Are those for whom some form of behavior control is deemed necessary capable of granting consent for such invasions of their psyche or brain? Should prisoners be required to grant consent for participation in rehabilitative programs, when they obviously do not give consent to be incarcerated in the first place?

Therapy or Social Control

With this list of questions as background, we can now introduce the problem of distinguishing therapy from social control, to which we shall return later. It is obvious that the same techniques can be used for the purpose of therapy (trying to cure or improve the ill person's condition) or for the purpose of social control (trying to bring about conformity with society's norms and laws). Both may well be legitimate purposes. Among the examples in which the distinction becomes hard to make are the use of Ritalin hydrochloride or amphetamines on hyperactive school-children and the use of psychosurgery on both mental patients and prisoners. Further examples include the present behavior-modification programs for inmates and the proposed use of experimental drugs on imprisoned sex offenders, as well as more ordinary psychotherapeutic techniques such as group therapy, Gestalt therapy, or even traditional talk therapy frequently used to help manage institutionalized persons. It may turn out that what is permissible under the guise of therapy is not permissible under the guise of social control. The trick is to sort out, if possible, when the case is one of therapy and when it is an instance of social control. Psychosurgery, chemical agents, and electrical stimulation of the brain can be used to cure or improve the condition or they can be used as means of social control, inside or outside institutions like prisons or mental hospitals. Whether a particular form of intervention can be justified as a means of therapy or as a mode of social control depends partly on the purposes of the behavior changers, partly on the setting in which the change is made (hospitals, prisons, or elementary schools), but mostly on other factors more germane to morality: whether fundamental rights are violated, whether the best interest of the entire community is served, whether the freedom and privacy of individuals should prevail over the welfare of the whole. The study of the ethics of behavior control thus requires a look at facts, theories, concepts, and principles.

Conflict Between Moral Values

Ethical dilemmas arise when there is a conflict of values, when two or more moral principles clash in situations in which both cannot be followed simultaneously. In modern Western culture, we generally believe that we have an obligation to respect other people's autonomy, and refrain from interfering with their basic freedom. But we also think it a good thing to promote people's well-being and to prevent unnecessary harm from befalling them—forms of interference often labeled "paternalism." But what are the practical implications of these moral beliefs? Does it mean that adults should or should not be allowed free access to mood-altering drugs, be they heroin, amphetamines, or tranquilizers, when the only persons likely to be harmed are the drug users themselves? Should suicidal persons be confined against their wishes—"For their own good"—when psychiatrists judge the likelihood of a suicide attempt to be high? These are only two of many examples in which paternalism and respect for autonomy come into conflict with one another in social policy settings.

The Main Features of Ethical Concerns

At least two main features serve to mark off ethical concerns from other concerns. First, people usually hold ethics to be very important in private and public life, especially when they feel they have been wronged in some way. Often, but not always, the moral considerations are thought to override others when hard decisions have to be made. Some philosophers argue that in those cases in which moral considerations are *not* viewed as overriding, they nevertheless ought to be so viewed. These philosophers might also claim that the failure to see moral considerations as having overarching value is a mark of moral blindness, moral weakness, or callousness.

The second chief feature of ethical situations is that they almost always seem to involve human interactions—what people do to or for other people. Though with the rise of animal liberation, some argue that the domain of ethics should be widened to include animals—at least those reasonably high on the phylogenetic scale. Even in earlier centuries, moral philosophers such as John Stuart Mill expressed concern for the treatment of animals by including all sentient creatures among those whose interests must be considered when deciding which courses of action are morally permissible or desirable. But for the most part, worries about ethics relate to human beings.

It should be apparent how the second core element of ethics is closely linked with controlling or trying to alter human behavior. The subjects of ethical concern are human beings—all of us in ordinary society, as well as the special populations on which much of this book focuses: psychiatric patients, the mentally retarded, prisoners, and others who obviously do not conform with—who deviate from—society's norms. It needs little reminder that policies and actions affecting such people are generally felt to be very important. Heated debates continue over the desirability and ethical permissibility of capital punishment. Lengthy testimony has been offered before congressional subcommittees on the subject of psychosurgery. And the entire practice—as well as specific details—of involuntary commitment remains a hot issue. When public opinion is sharply divided, when judges in different jurisdictions hand down decisions that conflict with one another, and when research on human violence and aggression is halted because of public or private opposition, there is a good chance that moral issues lurk nearby.

The reasons why individuals and interest groups lock horns on these issues are often political as well as moral, and they cannot always be easily distinguished from one another. People see themselves as having interests they want to preserve, and special-interest groups understandably try to maintain their power or get what they take to be their due. So it often happens that conflicts over issues of behavior control include both ethical and political factors, especially when the concept of justice enters in. The social climate of the times must also be taken into account in analyzing and drawing conclusions about the ethics of behavior control. In eras before dehumanizing "total institutions" were fashioned, there could be no debate about their mode of operation, whether they ought to be abolished, or what should be done with the "deinstitutionalized" former inmates. But in the present social system, policies need to be reevaluated in light of existing technical capabilities and changing social norms.

Means and Ends

In philosophical theory, as in everyday life, conflicts of value can occur either in choosing the means to whatever ends we have in mind, or in selecting the ends themselves. For example, everyone might agree on the desirability of the social goal of reducing violent crimes against people or on the need to protect people against abuses or violations of their rights by those in power. But when it comes to deciding what means are permissible for trying to bring about these agreed-upon ends, a storm of controversy erupts.

Some argue that punishment should be more severe or that sentences should be stricter for criminal offenders or that parole ought to be abolished. Making sure that criminals are securely behind bars is the appropriate means to the desired end: reducing violence against people.

Others, however, stress the need for further research on violence, arguing that incarcerating criminals does serve to keep those particular individuals off the streets, but what is needed most is more scientific research on the root causes of violence in order to gain better predictive and preventive measures. Those who urge greater research efforts also seek ways to control or even change the behavior of persons known or likely to be violent.

But there is considerable opposition to both of these proposed means of trying to reach an agreed-upon end. Opponents of the first proposal argue that passing harsher laws or using stricter sentencing practices would further worsen an already inhumane penal system—one that dehumanizes and degrades those unfortunates who have been led to commit antisocial acts. Opponents of the second proposal charge that research on human violence is often "mischievous" research. Moreover, even if the results of such research were to be helpful, such investigations could only be conducted on prisoners, who, according to some critics, cannot meaningfully grant consent to serve as research subjects. Whichever side opponents take and whatever policy decisions are made or laws enacted, these disputes focus mostly on what is morally permissible as a *means* to a generally desired social *end:* safety, security, and well-being in teeming urban centers and in the nation as a whole.

Debates also persist over which ends ought to be pursued, since it may not be possible to reach all desirable goals simultaneously. A system that brings maximum liberty to all individuals must usually sacrifice equality, and a society that strives for efficiency may do so at the expense of both liberty and equality.

The Role of Moral Philosophy

How can moral philosophy help in understanding and analyzing ethical problems and in deciding what ought to be done? Wherever there are efforts to control behavior, and whatever form these methods take, the use of techniques for altering people's behavior demands a defense in terms of good reasons. This is because our culture holds in high regard the values of individual liberty, privacy, and autonomy. Yet the reasons used to justify acts or practices accepted without question by some may, for their opponents, be the same reasons used to question the morality of certain types of behavior control. For example, those who see the necessity for the effectiveness of a technique might favor psychosurgery or electrode implantation in the brain rather than the less invasive—but also less effective—methods such as behavior modification or talk therapy. Those who place high value on rationality and autonomy are likely to choose modes of psychotherapy that emphasize self-understanding and conscious efforts at self-control.

The Problem of Establishing Moral Principles

Whether it is morally right to invade people's private lives by imposing changes on their thoughts, feelings, or actions—assuming it to be technically possible—depends on still other particular factors: the nature and characteristics of the subject; the motives, roles, and authority of those who exercise the control; and how much and in what ways other people are affected by the subject's past or present behavior. Are they really harmed? Or are they simply offended?

Is the safety of innocent family members and neighbors to be valued more than the liberty of a person who has committed no violent act but has been judged "dangerous to others"? And what if a person has made a suicide attempt and is judged "dangerous to self"? What moral principle should override respect for personal autonomy—the right of people to determine what they want and to act accordingly, in what concerns only themselves? Should it, perhaps, be the welfare of society or the state as a whole? Arguing consistently for or against the moral rightness of different forms of behavior control in a variety of circumstances requires, at some point, arguing for some moral principles.

Even knowing all these things is still not enough for putting together a moral theory about the scope and limits of behavior control. Ultimately, nothing short of a comprehensive theory, linking psychological and ethical precepts, will do. Only then can rational and consistent answers be provided for specific moral problems in the practice of psychiatry, the criminal justice system, the schools, or in any institution whose inmates require management in some form. But to have a moral theory, what is needed first and foremost are secure moral principles. Here, as always, is where the trouble will lie: in choosing an undisputed set of principles to form the heart of the theory.

Behavior Control as Public Policy

This book will explore the chief ethical issues in behavior control by discussing several prominent moral principles and basic ethical concepts. Much of the discussion will focus on efforts to control behavior in institutions—hospitals, prisons, research centers, and schools. This special focus is not meant to ignore private psychiatry or the other areas where behavior control is practiced—organized religion, industry and labor, and the family. But since any study must limit its scope, the limiting principle for this book will be a focus on the ethics of behavior control as it raises issues of public policy, rather than of private practice in psychiatry or clinical psychology. Accordingly, the behavior-control methods and technologies that will be cited most are the use of psychoactive drugs; psychosurgery; electrical stimulation of the brain (ESB) by means of electrode implantation; electroconvulsive therapy (ECT—more commonly known as shock treatment); and institutional programs using techniques such as behavior modification, which employs positive reinforcements (rewards) or aversive stimuli (punishments).

Certainly, the behavior or personality, or both, of more people have been changed by converting to an Eastern religion, by enrolling in courses in assertiveness training, or by embracing cults like EST or Scientology than by psychosurgery. These other efforts at behavior control also raise serious issues of public policy, often similar to those provoked by the newest developments in psychopharmacology, behavioral conditioning, or increasingly refined techniques of neurosurgery. Yet there are differences. Ethical issues dealing with cults are largely tied to religious freedom, and conceptual concerns become entangled in the somewhat dubious appeal to "brainwashing." Both the institutional context in which technological interventions are used, and the fact that they invade normally inviolable rights of privacy make these ethical issues matters of more widespread legal, social, and political importance. As policy issues, they deserve center stage. As matters for ethical inquiry, modes of behavior control promoted by psychiatrists, psychologists, educators, and administrators, and sanctioned by the state, force a reexamination of the concept of freedom and related concepts such as responsibility, autonomy, coercion, paternalism, competence, rationality, and voluntariness.

It is beyond the scope of this study to explore in detail each of these fundamental ethical notions. But it is worth recalling that traditional and contemporary moral philosophy has produced a wealth of theories and analyses of those concepts, and it may be helpful to begin by making some fundamental distinctions before plunging into the thicket of complex issues surrounding the question: Who may do what to whom, and with what justification?

Behavior Control: Theory and Applications

Methods used to control behavior are not chosen out of thin air. Rather, they are almost always linked to some theory that explains why these methods work as they do and also that is able to predict to some extent. Sometimes the specific mechanisms are unknown, and so a precise explanation of why a method works as it does is lacking. This is true for many drugs, as well as for the still widely used electric shock therapy for mental patients who respond to no other treatment. But even where gaps in knowledge occur, a general scientific framework exists. As more is learned through experiments or clinical trials, details continue to be filled in.

Before the scientific advances leading to today's sophisticated knowledge of brain physiology and anatomy and biochemical mechanisms of the body, human action and the efforts to control it were for the most part described in terms of behavior. Homespun adages such as "spare the rod and spoil the child" reflect a commonsense theory about the relationship between corporal punishment (or the lack of it) and character development. Homespun adages do not amount to a psychological theory, of course, but more detailed studies of human motivation and development should have something to say about the effect of beatings as a form of punishment on children's future behavior and personality.

Self-Control

Psychological theories attempt to explain why people think, feel, and act the way they do. But it is not only the control of one person's behavior by another that such theories try to explain. *Self*-control also needs explaining. What are the psychological causes of self-control? Why do some people have it while others lack it? How can it best be developed in the young? Control of one's own behavior must surely be thought of as part of the larger domain of behavior control. This is in part because people learn to control their own behavior in the same sorts of ways that the behavior of others is controlled. One feature of self-control is the ability to delay gratification. For example, the student who postpones partying with friends until his or her term paper is finished not only demonstrates the ability to delay gratification but also positively reinforces good study habits by rewarding the desired end: the completion of work. Behaviorist learning theory has shown that this increases the likelihood of such behavior patterns in the future.

Beyond that, a value component is embedded in the notion of self-control. Whatever the disagreement over the ethics of behavior control by the state or by psychiatric practices in prisons and mental hospitals, there appears to be widespread agreement about the positive value of self-control. Most people think it a good thing to remain in command of their actions, not to let themselves get out of control in dealing with life's hardships.

Yet people obviously differ over the question of where self-control ends and being compulsive or "uptight" begins. The young mother who cannot enjoy a good novel while her children nap because she has to scour the bathroom; the executive who cannot leave the office before 7:30 P.M. because she must answer all of today's correspondence; the professor who is committed to grading students' papers by the end of the weekend, resulting in a refusal to join a Sunday family outing: These examples may be described both as exercises in self-control, and as instances of compulsive behavior. Which description is the "correct" one depends more on matters of personal taste or social norms than on objective moral principles. Matters of taste are usually called "subjective" values; moral principles have an objectivity that goes beyond the personal values people happen to hold, and thus they demand wider adherence. Personality theories in psychology and psychiatry approach the topic of self-control as part of the larger domain of behavior control. This usually takes the form of a theory of motivation. But for the most part, such theories remain silent on the value issues described in these examples.

Understanding Human Behavior

A theory of human personality must underlie every behavior-control program or practice. In order to know what is likely to be effective and why, there needs to be a systematic approach that links efforts to control human behavior with an explanatory theory. The aims of science are explanation, prediction, and control. A fully worked out, well-confirmed scientific theory should provide an explanation for events that are the objects of study, offer a reliable basis for prediction, and suggest a framework on which to devise means of control. When the object of control is human behavior, ethical issues cannot lag far behind.

But even among scientific theories that now compete in attempting to explain and predict human behavior, debate and controversy continue to rage among different schools of thought. To cite only one example, orthodox behaviorist theory has no need for, and explicitly rejects, explanations of behavior that appeal to mental states, intrapsychic forces, or irreducible emotional or cognitive states. The only elements needed—or even tolerated—in a scientific psychology are bits of outward behavior or observable behavior patterns. In contrast, an essential feature of psychoanalytic theory is that the elements used to explain human actions cannot be merely behavioral; all overt acts and behavioral traits must be explained by *motives*, couched in terms of psychodynamic or developmental forces. This is only one difference between these two theories; and still other schools of theory and practice, such as existential psychiatry and humanistic psychology, take an altogether different approach. The latter theories reject the view that scientific determinism offers the only possible explanatory mode for human behavior. Existentialist approaches hold a conception of human agents as creatures having free will, in contrast to other views maintaining that a scientific psychology must be able to give causal explanations of behavior it seeks to change. These and other psychological theories are "competing" in the sense that they all strive to offer the "correct" explanation, and also to be most accurate and effective in achieving the scientific aims of prediction and control.

Different Kinds of Dispute

A great many disputes are a mix of conceptual, scientific, and philosophical arguments. To take only one example, one strong criticism of leading forms of therapy is that they are simply ineffective as methods of behavior change. Behavioral psychologists have been saying for years that "psychoanalysis doesn't work," or when it does, it is unnecessarily long and drawn out. Others charge that doing nothing at all about neurotic disturbances gets the same results as doing something—whatever that something is. Still others—opponents of the behaviorist approach—hold that operant conditioning (the mode of therapy using positive reinforcement) is not as effective as behaviorists would have us believe. One thing missing from these general criticisms is a clear indication of what criteria are used to determine effectiveness. Another way of stating the point is that there is often no clear definition of "effective"; and opponents in the debate do not always use the chief concepts—"effectiveness," "results," "what works"—in the same sense. These are among the conceptual difficulties in this case.

There is also empirical disagreement—disagreement over the facts. One charge is that behavior modification may work very well in changing tiny bits of behavior like fingernail biting or facial twitches, but it fails when it comes to larger patterns of human behavior. Behaviorists might disagree by pointing to their results: Cases can be found in which wide-ranging patterns of unwanted behavior underwent significant changes. If the facts are uncontested but the disagreement remains, this is probably a clue that the disagreement is either conceptual or moral, and concerns "significance" or "wide-ranging behavior patterns." Effectiveness and efficiency are values that remain at the heart of debates surrounding the merits of different behavior-control methods, although other moral concerns are deeper and weigh more importantly in the end.

To get embroiled in such debates would require much more analysis and statistical inquiry than this study allows. It would be necessary to examine the notion of "success" used in judgments that behavior-modification techniques, such as positive reinforcements to reward desired behavior, are far more successful than psychoanalysis. Usually, those who favor behavior modification emphasize the effectiveness and efficiency of this method over the various "talk" therapies. Promoters of psychoanalytic therapy have what behaviorists consider a standard answer. Since such replies are based on a belief in inner, psychodynamic mechanisms—a belief rejected by behaviorists—there is no way in principle of settling the dispute. What is needed is a criterion for "success," specifying the type of behavior or emotion—its scope and depth—that has undergone change as a result of therapy. One question for the behaviorists is how long can the specific behavioral change last. Can the desired ("corrected") behavior be maintained without continuing positive reinforcements? If not, should the therapy be counted as successful? Many conceptual and theoretical questions deserve deeper examination. These questions raise doubts even about what should count as change in behavior, personality, or feelings.

Add to these ongoing disputes all the disagreements about moral matters, and it is no wonder that the field of behavior control is rich with ethical issues. We shall be skirting most of the theoretical concerns relating to explanation and prediction of human behavior, but not because such concerns are uninteresting or unimportant. At least some questions of ethics may be laid to rest by gains in knowledge or the settlement of disputes over matters of scientific fact or theory. Although techniques of behavior control involving physical alteration of the brain or alteration of mood by powerful chemicals are the ones most likely to provoke concern about their use or abuse, the even less dramatic forms of intervention like psychotherapy and behavior modification—which use no chemicals, electrodes, or surgical tools— raise moral issues.

Worries About Behavior Control

What is it that all these methods have in common, causing concerns and fears about their use on particular individuals or groups—mental patients, prisoners, children, or research subjects? Is it that they all use sophisticated technology instead of the more "natural" methods of behavior control used for centuries in everyday life? Is it that we may suspect the motives of those in charge of ordering or administering the techniques? Does the chief problem stem from the fact that adult human beings have fundamental rights of privacy that prohibit us from interfering with their behavior or personality, no matter how benevolent may be the motives of those in power or authority?

Perhaps it is the wrong approach to ask which *forms* of intervention aimed at behavior control are morally permissible and which are not. The resolution of such ethical dilemmas may not depend on which particular therapeutic technique or behavior control technology is used but on something else. At first, it may seem that the more a technique invades the body or the mind, the greater the probability that ethical problems will emerge, and that, in the whole range of behavior control methods, the "hard" methods intuitively seem more coercive and hence unacceptable. At the "hard" end of the spectrum lie psychosurgery and other forms of physical manipulation of the brain; the "soft" methods of influencing behavior include propaganda, advertising, and the traditional forms of education used in the classroom or at home. But whether a technique is "hard" or "soft" may well turn out to be less morally relevant than it seems at first. For example, among the morally significant factors is whether or not the subject has granted—or is capable of granting—voluntary, informed consent for the procedure, whatever qualities it possesses.

It is worth keeping separate two different lines along which a continuum might be drawn. One marks off the different types of physical or psychological intervention, ranging from the most invasive or intrusive procedure to the mildest. The other continuum is a conceptual one that relates more directly to ethics: extreme coercion and punishment lie at one end and mild inducements or attractive rewards at the other. Along this conceptual continuum, the so-called gunman model ("your money or your life") may seem to present the most coercive threat, since although there appears to be a choice presented to the victim, it is a forced choice. The gunman controls the behavior of the victim by making an offer he cannot refuse. It is merely an ironic use of the term to say that the person threatened under the gunman model has a "choice" between two courses of action.

It has become fashionable lately to refer to almost any enticement, inducement, or form of persuasion as "coercive." But it is important to sort out these different notions clearly, lest we be unable to distinguish those offers people cannot (psychologically) refuse from those they can resist by efforts of the will or can become able to resist if they achieve conscious awareness of what is going on. In one area of current debate, failure to distinguish carefully among coercion, manipulation, enticements, inducements, and incentives is one factor contributing to the confusion about the ethics of using prisoners as research subjects. A chief point of controversy is whether prisoners are capable of granting fully voluntary consent because of the "inherently coercive environment" in which they dwell. But is it accurate to call the environment itself "coercive"? It is probably better to restrict the concept to actions performed by one human being against another for the purpose of control, for protection, or for self-defense in order to get a clear picture of what is at stake in ethical dilemmas over behavior control.

The Conceptual Continuum

Coercion

To fix ideas about the elements along the conceptual spectrum, ranging from coercion to the weakest modes of influence, consider these somewhat loose definitions. On the "gunman model," *coercion* always involves a threat of force or bodily harm by one person against another or against another's relative—a child, for example. The purpose of the coercer is to get the person coerced to do what the coercer wishes him or her to do—something that person would not otherwise do voluntarily and intentionally. On this account, a threat of force is always an element in coercive situations; for this reason we can keep them conceptually distinct from other forms of influence that have the effect of controlling behavior.

There is much debate, however, over whether merely offering people things they cannot (psychologically) refuse should properly be considered a form of coercion, when no threat of force or bodily harm is involved. Is an offer of five million dollars to commit a petty crime coercive? Is an offer of job promotion to a rising young executive, a grade of A to a premedical student, or a presidential cabinet appointment to an ambitious politician coercive, if the offer is made to secure some favor or as a promised reward for cooperating? Such acts are often termed "coercive," although they lack the element of force. To keep the language clear, it would be best to restrict the term "coercion" to those acts directly involving threats of force and to use the term "manipulation" for non-force situations. When someone makes generous offers of material goods or higher status in return for a favor it might appropriately be called manipulation.

Manipulation

But making generous offers is not the only way of manipulating people into doing what you want them to do; there is another, even better-known, method of behavior control in ordinary life. That form of manipulation takes place when one person deceives another in order to gain something for himself. Some kinds of deception are intended to help the person deceived: lying for benevolent motives (the white lie) or deceiving children to protect them from information they can't handle. But selfish or egoistic lies are motivated by the deceiver's perception of his own interests.

To *manipulate* people is to "handle them," a figurative image calling to mind the way a puppeteer pulls the strings of his marionettes. That people are not mere marionettes is clear, in spite of the apparent implications of psychic determinism. Marionettes are simple creations and therefore not comparable to humans with their biological and psychological complexity. That humans are not "organic computers" is a much more difficult hypothesis to attempt to refute. But the puppet image is a useful one, particularly in two situations: when the subjects of manipulation are especially weak or dependent and when they are in a situation in which they are more vulnerable than they would normally be—as in a prison, hospital, school, or other institutional setting. While manipulative acts might appropriately be termed "coercion," it is best to keep distinctly separate those cases in which people may have some reasonable alternative course of action and those like the gunman example, in which they may suffer physical harm or even death if they fail to comply.

Seduction, temptation

Weaker still than manipulation is *seduction* or *temptation*—offering people pleasures or goods they would like to have, but they do not experience such an overwhelming response that they can do nothing but accept. People who readily give in to seductions or temptations are often described as suffering from "weakness of the will." The language may be quaint, but it suggests an important link between moral and psychological concepts. A person whose will is weak—who readily gives in to temptations—is generally held morally responsible and open to blame for backsliding from acceptable social behavior. Contrast this with the two preceding categories of action: doing what someone else wishes because of a threat of force (coercion) and doing what someone else wishes because of offers of great sums of money or positions of power and prestige (manipulation). Experience makes it clear why so many people give in to temptations or seductions in some form, at one time or other, and so perform acts they otherwise would not freely choose to do. But such acts are not made ethically acceptable by the mere fact that we understand why people perform them. Further justification is needed to excuse a person who acts wrongly as a result of being sorely tempted.

Persuasion

Moving along the continuum from most coercive to least coercive, we come next to the concept of *persuasion*. Acts of persuasion often begin with the presumption that the persons to be persuaded stand roughly on an equal footing in both reason and power with those using the persuasive techniques. The techniques may include reason, argument, and entreaty. Propaganda, too, is a mode of persuasion. But to the extent that propaganda or advertising uses deceit or fraud, it is more like manipulation than like persuasion. These categories are not perfectly clear and distinct, since acts of persuasion that proceed by reasoning are surely different in method and effect from persuasive techniques that appeal to the hearers' emotions. The next chapter will explore this topic more fully in examining the distinction between behavior-control techniques that bypass the rational processes and those that employ them.

Indoctrination; education

Distinguishing between the rational and the nonrational is also important in another pair of concepts. There is probably no sharp line between *indoctrination* and the somewhat weaker notion of *education*. The process of educating usually involves activities (for example, role-modeling) that go beyond the mere giving of information. More important, however, is the development of critical skills, which requires an ability to reason soundly. This difference between the methods of education and those of indoctrination may lie in the form of instruction, in the intentions of teachers versus indoctrinators, or in the setting—for example, a retreat run by members of a cult as opposed to a public school where cultural and religious differences are supposed to be respected and tolerated. But indoctrination usually has other elements as well—elements of persuasion, especially those that appeal to emotions or attitudes. A special mode of indoctrination is the form of behavior control known as "thought reform" or "brainwashing." These terms lack a clear, objective meaning, and mental health professionals are puzzled over whether or not the terms actually refer to some special psychological phenomenon, and if so, what it is. Different settings in which brainwashing is said to have occurred have a number of features in common: The victims are prisoners or captives, such as prisoners of war in Korea or Vietnam; or they were manipulated or enticed into joining a single-purpose group, such as the Moonies, in which leaders use extreme emotional arousal of subjects and cut them off almost totally, psychologically and socially, from their previous supports—family, friends, religion, or other ideological commitments. Similarities between the methods of behavior control used by religious cults and those employed by political or ideological groups are described by one scholar as follows:

> The persuader and his group represent a comprehensive and pervasive world view, which incorporates supremely powerful suprapersonal forces. That communism identifies these forces with the Party, while religions regard them as supernatural is

relatively unimportant for the purpose of this discussion. The world view is infallible and cannot be shaken by the sufferer's failure to change or improve. The suprapersonal powers are contingently benevolent; the sufferer may succeed in obtaining their favor if he shows the right attitude. . . .

The means by which changes in the sufferer are brought about include a particular type of relationship and some sort of systematic activity or ritual. . . . The systematic activity characteristically involves means of emotional arousal, often to the point of exhaustion, leading to an altered state of consciousness that increases susceptibility to outside influences.[1]

Whether these methods of behavior control are called "brainwashing," "thought reform," or simply "indoctrination," they differ fundamentally from education in the role that reason plays in education but not in indoctrination. Yet education has another quality that makes it a powerful mode of behavior control: its lasting effect on the way people think and act. As Plato pointed out in *The Republic*, the process of education is among the most effective means of shaping later behavior, particularly when the learners are still at an impressionable age.

The Technological Spectrum

Psychosurgery

Let us turn now to the technological spectrum ranging from the most intrusive or "hardest" to the least intrusive, or "softest," methods of behavior control. Consider, first, the one usually considered the most invasive method of all: *psychosurgery*. A recent book describing the history of psychosurgery recounts one now-discarded technique of frontal lobotomy in these terms:

In 1942 Walter Freeman, a neurologist, and James Watts, a neurosurgeon, . . . reported that extreme depression and agitation—even hallucinations— could be greatly alleviated by cutting the fibers leading from the frontal lobe of the brain to the neighboring thalamus. . . . After cutting these connections, the doctors reported that exaggerated emotion responses decreased. . . .

The Freeman-Watts treatment spread quickly, and during the 1940s somewhere in the range of fifty thousand patients were lobotomized in the United States alone. Dr. Freeman was a lobotomy zealot and calculated that he had personally performed more than 3500 operations, using a gold-plated icepick which he carried with him in a velvet-lined case. After the local application of a mild pain-killer, Dr. Freeman would plunge the icepick through the thin bone of the upper inner angle of the eye socket, severing the frontal nerve connections to the thalamus. No elaborate preparations or precautions preceded this grisly operation, which often took place in the patient's home or in Dr. Freeman's office. . . . [2]

More recently developed, highly refined techniques of psychosurgery are vastly different from the accurately named "icepick method" that was hotly debated for several decades. Not only was the earlier technique a crude one, which involved cutting of normal tissue, but its effects on the entire personality were almost always

[1] Jerome D. Frank, *Persuasion and Healing* (New York: Schocken Books, 1974), pp. 103–4.

[2] Richard M. Restak, *Pre-meditated Man* (New York: Viking Press, 1973), pp. 5–6.

devastating. The classical "frontal lobe syndrome" included loss of initiative, inappropriate joviality, and social insensitivity.[3]

Again in the last few years, the battle over the merits and risks of psychosurgery has revived. In an article discussing a landmark court case *(Kaimowitz* v. *Department of Mental Health)* on the proposed use of psychosurgery on a prisoner, the author writes: "Psychosurgery is the most drastic means of affecting human behavior. It produces an immediate, extensive and irreversible change in the subject's personality; it requires a physical intrusion into the brain; it is impossible for a subject to resist."[4]

Patients who have undergone one of the newer, more precise forms of psychosurgery come out of the operating room looking and acting very different from the image portrayed in print and on stage and screen in *One Flew Over the Cuckoo's Nest*. New knowledge about the structure and function of the human brain, as well as technological advances in neuroscience, make possible careful diagnosis and precision surgery by means of three-dimensional brain-scanning devices. One of the surgical techniques that have replaced the old frontal lobotomy is know as "prefrontal leucotomy," and another is called "cingulotomy." Leucotomy has been used on patients "selected for surgery because of severe levels of anxiety, depression, or obsessionality which were unresponsive to all other appropriate modes of treatment."[5] These methods were further refined into specialized techniques of subcortical leucotomy: "leucotomy of the lateral frontal area was used for patients with paranoid delusions; orbital subcortical lesions were used for anxious patients; and mesial leucotomy was used for aggresive patients."[6] Sterotactic cingulotomy has also been used to treat patients with a number of aggressive conditions and has been reported to have significant benefits to some. Cingulotomy has been praised as a treatment for depression and obsessive-compulsive disorders, as well as schizophrenia.

These and other techniques of neurological surgery are scientifically respectable and are not considered unethical when there is a tumor or other evidence of brain pathology or injury. The destruction of normal tissue only because of deviant behavior, however, poses moral problems.

Psychosurgery, raises questions of law and policy, especially when performed on persons who are aggressive or violent. The meaning of aggression and violence depends largely on the social setting in which they occur. Because many psychologists and psychiatrists are convinced that social and political factors help cause people to become violent, they consider it a mistake to focus intervention primarily on the brain. Exactly what is "aggressive" or "violent" behavior? Peaceable

[3]Herbert G. Vaughan, Jr., "Psychosurgery and Brain Stimulation in Historical Perspective," in Willard M. Gaylin, Joel S. Meister, and Robert Neville (eds.), *Operating on the Mind* (New York: Basic Books, 1975), p. 42. For a full discussion of the ethical, legal, and policy issues concerning psychosurgery, see the other essays in this volume.

[4]Jay Alexander Gold, "Kaimowitz v. Department of Mental Health: Involuntary Mental Patient Cannot Give Informed Consent to Experimental Psychosurgery," *New York University Review of Law and Social Change,* IV (Spring 1974), p. 207.

[5]J. S. Smith, L. G. Kiloh, and J. A. Boots, "Prospective Evaluation of Prefrontal Leucotomy: Results in 30 Months' Followup," in *Neurosurgical Treatment in Psychiatry, Pain, and Epilepsy,* eds. W. H. Sweet, S. Obrador, and J. C. Martín-Rodríguez (Baltimore: University Park Press, 1977), p. 217.

[6]R. Saubidet, J. Lyonnet, and D. Brichetti, "Undercutting of Lateral Aspect of Frontal Lobes for Treatment in the Chronic Paranoid Psychosis, Paraphrenia," in Sweet, Obrador, and Martín-Rodríguez, p. 225.

antiwar demonstrations? Passive resistance to gain political ends? A value bias may enter into judgments of violence or aggression. The use of surgery to "cure" such behavior patterns has been blamed for contributing to the "medicalization" of deviant forms of behavior. This is one example of the increasing compass of the medical model.

No matter how precise and elegant the techniques of psychosurgery may become, the basic moral issues remain open for debate. These issues include at least the following concerns: the difficulty of assessing accurately the risks against the benefits of psychosurgical procedures; the question of whether a candidate for psychosurgery is capable of granting voluntary, informed consent; whether physical manipulation of the brain is really an invasion of a person's privacy; and the likelihood that those who have decision-making power will abuse such procedures.

What is the basis for ethical objections to psychosurgery? Some objections stem from a philosophical theory about the nature of persons—a conceptual analysis or metaphysical account of what human beings "really are." In this argument against the practice of psychosurgery, the irreversibility or permanence of its effects is all important. For instance, versions of the mind-body theory known as physicalism or materialism (the view that people are made of the same stuff as the rest of the universe), in particular the "neural identity theory," generally hold that the brain constitutes the "core person"; it would follow that its change by surgery destroys or deforms that person. Many people share the view that to invade the (normal) brain is to intrude on the person in fundamental ways—ways that may be morally questionable even when the subject signs a consent form or expresses a strong desire to have his or her brain manipulated by certain behavior-control techniques. If the person has psychological impairment, the problem is most acute, since competency to grant consent requires rational understanding and the ability to exercise free choice. As it was put in a hearing on psychosurgery before a U.S. Senate subcommittee, "the damaged organ is the consenting organ."[7]

But as usual in ethical arguments, there are two sides to the story. One side queries: "If a person freely and knowingly requests or consents to procedures that alter basic thinking processes, moods, or values, and especially when those changes are desirable ones, what could be ethically wrong with granting such a request?" The other side replies: "The sorts of changes that might be wrought are ones that even a rational person could not, in principle, be able to know about in advance. If the behavior or character change is widespread enough or deep enough, a different person (in the sense of personality) may emerge. This goes beyond the point where consent can be truly informed." Whether or not that claim is true, there remains the problem of whether someone caught in the grip of mental illness can, in principle, freely consent to psychosurgery or other behavior-altering procedures.

Once the notion of granting informed consent enters the picture, the ethical issues posed by psychosurgery are no longer unique. Not all behavior-control technologies involving physical manipulation of the brain are irreversible like psychosurgery. But difficulties in obtaining fully informed, voluntary consent are one issue; those that stem from the permanence or scope of the effects are another concern. Positive as well as negative results of psychosurgery are cited in the ongoing debate, and it is probably true that patients have benefitted from this technique when all other therapies had failed. One side argues that since some

---

[7]Willard Gaylin, testimony before the Subcommittee on Health of the Senate Committee on Labor and Public Welfare, 93rd Cong., 1st sess. (1973).

patients have enjoyed these clear benefits, it would be unethical *not* to use them where conditions indicate that others could find relief from their suffering. Yet taken to its extreme, this view can become narrowly medical, as in this statement from a recent medical text on the subject: "Ultimately, the basic ethical problem of psychosurgery is only medical: whether psychosurgery can or cannot alleviate psychic illness without causing harmful side effects."[8] Judgments about which side effects are harmful, and how harmful such effects have to be before they outweigh the benefits, are not strictly "medical" problems. They raise value issues of a fundamental sort—issues that should be distinguished from the equally important conceptual and empirical issues also in need of analysis.

Electrical Stimulation

Various modes of *electrical stimulation* have been tested on primates, and some are already in use with human subjects. These include ESB (electrical stimulation of the brain), in which electrodes are inserted in the brain, and ECT (electroconvulsive therapy), better known among the general public as shock treatment. Paddles are placed outside the patient's head and electric current is transmitted through them. The specific forms ESB can take include the implantation of electrodes and electronic devices in the brains of subjects, which reveal their physical location as well as monitor their brain wave activity, and other highly refined electronic devices.

In an article entitled "Intracerebral Radio Stimulation and Recording in Completely Free Patients," Dr. José Delgado, one of the leaders in brain manipulation, describes in detail the diameter in millimeters of such devices, their electrical oscillation frequency, exactly where in the anatomical structure of the brain they are supposed to be inserted, as well as other features of such intracerebral electronic wizardry. Especially notable for its ethical implications is a three-channel unit for radio stimulation and EEG telemetry, which Delgado calls the "stimoceiver" (*stimulator* and EEG *receiver*). Discussing the experimental design for the research on that device, Delgado claims that "the purpose of this study was to identify sites of abnormal intracerebral activity and to test brain excitability in order to guide contemplated therapeutic surgery."[9] As a believer in psychosurgery as well as various modes of electrical intervention into the brain, Delgado is not troubled by the fact that some ESB methods are being developed for the purpose of helping make psychosurgery itself easier. In order not to mislead, however, it is important to note that more often, electronic forms of brain intervention are promoted or used because they serve as an *alternative* to surgical intervention. They also serve as an alternative of another sort: an alternative to imprisonment or to institutionalization of some types of mental patients.

Although these surgical and electronic techniques are now used mostly for therapy on patients who show abnormal brain-wave activity, they are being used experimentally and are being considered for people who only behave abnormally and have no signs of abnormal brain-wave activity. Many of these surgical and

---

[8]L. V. Laitinen, "Ethical Aspects of Psychiatric Surgery," in Sweet, Obrador, and Martín-Rodíguez, p. 487.

[9]José M. R. Delgado, "Intracerebral Radio Stimulation and Recording in Completely Free Patients," in *Psychotechnology: Electronic Control of Mind and Behavior,* eds. Robert L. Schwitzgebel and Ralph K. Schwitzgebel (New York: Holt, Rinehart and Winston, 1973), p. 188.

electronic procedures are still considered new, experimental forms of therapy, thus raising an additional ethical issue—the use of human subjects for biomedical and behavioral research.

Psychopharmocology

Having reviewed the surgical and electrical ways of controlling behavior, we come now to the third major means of altering actions and mood: the chemical way. There is little doubt that most research in *psychopharmacology* has been aimed at developing new drugs for therapeutic purposes. Yet the same techniques or substances available for therapeutic purposes can also be used for a different aim—as a method of social control. Since the psychopharmacological revolution began, after World War II, hundreds of drugs with a wide variety of effects on mood, thinking, and behavior have emerged. Because of their bearing on ethical issues in behavior control, three classes of drugs are worth describing briefly here.

The first category includes those mood-altering (psychotropic) substances known as antipsychotic drugs. The largest and most widely used group are the phenothiazines. Since these powerful chemicals are often used to make patients in psychiatric hospitals more "manageable," they are correctly described as agents of social control, as well as therapeutic agents. Yet sometimes manageability of the patient is a necessary first step before any therapy can be tried. Antipsychotic medications are also used for outpatients, who might otherwise have to remain institutionalized, and so these drugs provide an alternative to institutionalization for at least some severely disturbed people. The distinction between therapy and social control is none too clear. Nor is it evident how to balance the tradeoffs when mental patients are deinstitutionalized and kept on heavy doses of tranquilizing medication.

A second category of drugs includes the antiandrogens—chemicals that counteract male hormones. The best known of these is cyproterone acetate, which has been dubbed a form of "chemical castration." Antiandrogens are viewed as therapeutic agents for treatment of violent sex offenders. But if they succeed in their intended aim, this class of drugs can obviously be used for the purpose of social control. Here again, if offered to chronic sex offenders as an alternative to incarceration, the dual role of such drugs becomes apparent. Some find it ethically troubling simply to offer prisoners a choice between taking antiandrogens under ongoing medical supervision or remaining in prison indefinitely.

A third class of drugs are those used as aversive stimuli, almost always as part of a larger program of behavior modification. Perhaps the best known drug in this category is Antabuse, which has been used for years to combat alcoholism. Alcoholics in programs designed to combat alcoholism voluntarily consume this substance, which when combined with alcohol, produces violent bouts of nausea and vomiting. The pairing of this extremely unpleasant sensation with the otherwise pleasurable experience of drinking, often leads to "extinction" of the undesirable behavior. The idea behind its use in treatment programs is that one who is taking Antabuse has to make only one decision per day, which is much easier than many daily decisions not to drink. This method does not have a success rate of 100 percent, but neither does any other program to change behavior, in this category or any other.

Another drug—succinylcholine chloride (Anectine)—produces an extremely unpleasant sensation of drowning and suffocating. It has been paired with visual scenes or temptations leading to behavior that the patient, client, or prisoner wants (or is being "rehabilitated") to avoid. This is the classic "Clockwork Orange" method. Still other examples can be found among some of the drugs given to political prisoners in the Soviet Union. One of these is Haloperidol, a neuroleptic drug marketed in the United States as Haldol and used interchangeably with Thorazine as antipsychotic medication. In the Soviet Union, it

> is usually prescribed in cases of extreme "psychomotor excitation," and then usually with anti-Parkinsonian agents to counteract the painful and dangerous side effects. Given without counteracting agents, Haloperidol creates a hyperactive state in which the patient cannot be still—sitting, lying, or standing—for any period of time. It can also cause muscular spasms, stammering, involuntary contractions of the face and body and other symptoms associated with Parkinson's disease.[10]

A good example of the deliberate blurring of the distinction between therapy and social control thus appears to be the treatment of political dissidents in the U.S.S.R.

Education

It is fairly easy to see where ethical issues are likely to arise when the procedures used are invasive ones like psychosurgery, electrical stimulation of the brain, and powerful mood-altering drugs. But surprisingly reactions to the least invasive—the "softest"—methods of behavior control are equally strong. In the field of education, "textbook watching" has been gaining influence. Some people have become angered about the use of certain textbooks in public schools, especially books that teach evolutionary theory as being scientific truth, and others that present anthropological facts about values of people in other cultures.[11] There is also a long-standing debate over whether secular schools are the proper place to teach or preach moral values, or whether these subjects are not better confined to the home or to religious institutions. For some parents, what goes on in their children's schools has great moral import. Such controversies over compulsory prayers, religious observances, or even the use of science textbooks that explain the theory of evolution but fail to grant "equal time" to the biblical idea of creation become matters of principle. Often demands are made that new policies be instituted or old ones abandoned. But whatever the issue and whichever the interest group, many people firmly believe—as did Plato, almost 2500 years ago—that the role played by early education is dominant in shaping overall character as well as values. For those holding this belief, their children's elementary school education is a potentially dangerous form of behavior control, for both moral and psychological reasons. Parents who send their children to a military academy share this view, as do most parents who insist that their children go to strict denominational schools instead of attending free public schools.

Few claim to know, and even fewer agree on precisely to what extent the educational setting—if it could be separated from the influence of the home—could actually succeed in shaping behavior in fundamental ways. Lacking firm data, it is

---

[10]Ludmilla Thorne, "Inside Russia's Psychiatric Jails," *New York Times Magazine,* June 12, 1977, p. 27.

[11]Dorothy Nelkin, *Science Textbook Controversies and the Politics of Equal Time* (Boston: MIT Press, 1977).

risky to draw conclusions about what should be taught in public schools. There is little evidence that sex education, as usually offered in schools, does anything either to promote teenage pregnancy and venereal disease or to reduce the incidence of these conditions. Yet whether this subject should be in school curricula or not is rarely debated on the basis of empirical facts of this sort. Some parents remain vigorously opposed, while others rally in support, on the question of sex education in schools. Their commitment, one way or the other, seems based more on the values they hold than on evidence demonstrating that sex education, as usually taught, has any significant impact on the behavior or attitudes of adolescents.

These issues of behavior control naturally give rise to questions of policy. Decisions are made by principals, by school boards, by the state, or by whatever mechanisms are used to decide such matters. It is, in part, a debate over where the control should lie. Should it lie in the hands of the state, or should individuals enjoy maximum liberty and self-determination? The ethics of behavior control is through and through an inseparable mix of political, empirical, conceptual, theoretical, and moral questions.

FURTHER READINGS

BURGESS, ANTHONY, *A Clockwork Orange*. New York: Ballantine Books, 1976.
GOFFMAN, ERVING, *Asylums*. Garden City, N.Y.: Anchor Books, 1961.
KESEY, KEN, *One Flew Over the Cuckoo's Nest*. New York: Penguin, 1976.
LONDON, PERRY, *Behavior Control*. New York: New American Library (rev. ed.), 1977.
PLATO, *The Republic*.
SKINNER, B. F., *Beyond Freedom and Dignity*. New York: Alfred A. Knopf, 1972.

CHAPTER 2

Moral Philosophy and Behavior Control

Nature has placed mankind under the governance of two sovereign masters, *pain* and *pleasure*. It is for them alone to point out what we ought to do, as well as to determine what we shall do. On the one hand the standard of right and wrong, on the other the chain of causes and effects, are fastened to their throne. They govern us in all we do, in all we say, in all we think: every effort we can make to throw off our subjection, will serve but to demonstrate and confirm it. In words a man may pretend to abjure their empire: but in reality he will remain subject to it all the while. The *principle of utility* recognises this subjection, and assumes it for the foundation of that system, the object of which is to rear the fabric of felicity by the hands of reason and of law. Systems which attempt to question it, deal in sounds instead of sense, in caprice instead of reason, in darkness instead of light.

JEREMY BENTHAM
An Introduction to the Principles of Morals and Legislation

Everyone must admit that if a law is to have moral force, *i.e.*, to be the basis of an obligation, it must carry with it absolute necessity; that, for example, the precept, "Thou shalt not lie," is not valid for men alone, as if other rational beings had no need to observe it; and so with all the other moral laws properly so called; that, therefore, the basis of obligation must not be sought in the nature of man, or in the circumstances in the world in which he is placed, but *a priori* simply in the conceptions of pure reason; and although any other precept which is founded on principles of mere experience may be in certain respects universal, yet in as far as it rests even in the least degree on an empirical basis, perhaps only as to a motive, such a precept, while it may be a practical rule, can never be called a moral law.

IMMANUEL KANT
Fundamental Principles of the Metaphysic of Morals

The Issues

Despite many years of study and debate, philosophers or the general public have not agreed on which of many approaches to ethics is theoretically correct or most fruitful in practice. It is a mistake to think that moral philosophy can produce quick or easy solutions to the kinds of ethical problems sketched in the first chapter. Philosophers still continue to argue the merits of a number of competing ethical theories—utilitarian, libertarian, egalitarian, existentialist—each of which rests on some fundamental moral rule, principle, or approach. Some of these theories conflict directly with others. For example, the utilitarian conception of justice embodies the basic principle that it is morally permissible, under certain conditions, to interfere with people's liberty for the sake of the general welfare. More libertarian views assert an almost inviolable right of individual freedom, making it morally wrong ever to interfere with the behavior of any adults for their own good, and only in rare and extreme circumstances for the welfare of society as a whole. These two views come into direct conflict over this question: Under what conditions is it permissible to limit individual freedom? As a result, they will therefore come into direct conflict on some chief issues of behavior control.

These competing positions have their supporters in the world at large as well as among moral philosophers. Moral philosophy as a whole, then, cannot reasonably be expected to yield uncontroversial solutions to the ethical problems that plague society. So what can moral philosophy contribute toward resolving ethical quandaries related to the control of human behavior or toward making policy decisions in this area? For one thing, when practiced well, philosophy helps to make things clear, partly by sorting out a tangle of confused issues and partly by demanding that a position be stated cogently and precisely before it can be understood or accepted. Second, moral philosophy stands to contribute some fundamental principles, with reasons in support of them, which have developed within the Western tradition. Ethics is not, therefore, a merely subjective enterprise that can be reduced to the expression of the personal opinions and values of all who have something to say. There are objective standards for judging moral arguments and their conclusions, as well as for assessing policy decisions and their justifications.

Problems Arising from Psychological Theories

In addition to debates that continue to rage among theorists within philosophical ethics, the attempt to apply moral philosophy to the domain of behavior control poses special problems of its own. Many of these problems arise because of uncertainty and disagreement, even among experts, about the numerous methods and theories that populate the study of human behavior. What sort of explanation of human action is appropriate? One that specifies antecedent causes of behavior? One that rationalizes actions by focusing on the actor's own reasons? One that seeks to understand actions by examining the context in which they occur? What do various psychological theories tell us about the causes and control of human behavior? How can apparently conflicting theories be reconciled? What means of changing or shaping human behavior are most effective? How fixed are patterns of behavior once adulthood is reached?

These questions are primarily empirical and epistemological—matters of observation and understanding—addressed only secondarily to any values that may be attached. Questions about what *is* the case are factual questions. Questions about what *ought* to be the case are value questions. Obviously, not all value questions are of an ethical nature. Some involve esthetic judgments, others deal with economic values, still others merely express matters of taste, as in the preference for oysters over clams or a Mercedes over a Porsche.

Values and facts cannot always be clearly separated, although this point, too, remains under debate in contemporary philosophy. I agree with those who hold that there are conceptual as well as close causal ties between facts and values.[1] It is difficult, both in principle and in practice, to keep the two wholly separate. The term "sick," for example, imparts a (negative) value judgement, while it also purports to refer to a scientifically validated disease. When scientific, conceptual, and theoretical matters remain in dispute, in addition to the widespread differences that persist in the realm of moral values, these many difficulties have to be sorted out and addressed in turn. This is what is involved in the task of applying moral philosophy to practical concerns of behavior control. Given the present welter of theories in psychology and psychiatry—behaviorist, developmental, psychoanalytic, Gestalt, existential—it is not surprising that no clear agreement exists among professionals and practitioners in these fields about a large range of facts and concepts, to which any ethical theory must eventually be linked. To offer only one example, if the efforts to reform criminal offenders by using various psychological techniques are largely failures, this should have some implications for the continued use of the rehabilitative approach in penal institutions. Until there is much more agreement than now exists about what counts as success or failure, and which techniques work and which do not, a considerable degree of uncertainty will continue to accompany ethical debates in the sensitive area of behavior control.

"Ought Implies "Can"

In still further ways, the basic concerns of ethics are closely tied to psychological theories and their applications to human behavior. The concerns of ethics are with how people *ought* to act, not how they *do* or *will probably* act. Yet the latter is linked to the former. There is a well-known philosophical maxim that says: "Ought implies can." What this means is that before moral rules can reasonably be imposed on people, it must be possible, physically and psychologically, for those for whom the rules are intended to act in accord with them. Just as it is senseless to tell someone who seeks strenuous exercise that he ought to jump over the Empire State building, so too would it be pointless to tell people they ought to do something that is psychologically impossible. Freud criticized the commandment of Christian ethics, "Love thy neighbor as thyself," on this count. He writes:

> ... the cultural super-ego ... does not trouble itself enough about the facts of the mental constitution of human beings. It issues a command and does not ask whether it is possible for people to obey it. On the contrary, it assumes that a man's ego is psychologically capable of anything that is required of it, that his ego has unlimited mastery over his id.... The commandment, "Love thy neighbor as thyself," is an excellent example of the unpsychological proceedings of the cultural super-ego. The commandment is impossible to fulfill.... [2]

[1]For some examples of philosophical writings that argue in this vein, see: Philippa Foot, "Moral Beliefs," and John R. Searle, "How to Derive 'Ought' from 'Is'" in Philippa Foot (ed.), *Theories of Ethics* (Oxford: Oxford University Press, 1967).

[2]Sigmund Freud, *Civilization and its Discontents,* trans. and ed. by James Strachey (New York: W.W. Norton and Co., Inc., 1961), p. 90.

The basis for the "ought implies can" maxim lies in a consideration central to a number of key ethical issues in behavior control: people's responsibility for their actions. If the "ought implies can" precept is sound, the "can" part must be satisfied before it is appropriate to issue moral rules or judgments about what people ought to do. This is one area in which advances in the theory and practice of psychology and psychiatry are sorely needed. It is necessary to provide a clear, systematic account of human behavior—its explanation, prediction, and methods of control—in order to arrive at a conclusion about what is psychologically possible for people to do or to refrain from doing. The notion of psychological possibility has a philosophical counterpart in the idea of *freedom,* to which we turn next.

Two Concepts of Freedom

The concept most central to the ethics of behavior control is freedom. That notion is systematically ambiguous: It has two distinct, although related, meanings. The first is what is usually thought of as *political* liberty: individual freedom to pursue one's own ends or goals, with a minimum of outside interference from those in power—be they individuals or groups in society or officials of the state. The second meaning of "freedom" is the belabored notion of "free will," usually contrasted with psychic determinism, the view that all human thoughts, feelings, and actions are causally determined.

These two meanings of "freedom" should be kept separate, yet both bear on the ethics of behavior control. The sense of freedom associated with individual liberty refers to the degree and kind of unrestrained actions allowed to people, both in their behavior toward each other and also to themselves. In these latter cases—such as whether people ought to be allowed the freedom to take their own lives at will, or to have free access to drugs or other intoxicants that may harm only themselves—debate persists over the proper scope of state intervention. The distinction between "public" and "private" morality is central here. Should there be laws regulating the conduct of rational, consenting adults when there is no likely prospect of harm to others? Is government censorship of films, prohibition of sexual massage parlors, or regulation of homosexual activities justified? These questions need to be addressed in studying the proper role of government in regulating private conduct.

The second meaning of freedom is fundamentally metaphysical. It refers, not to freedom from interference by others or by the government, but rather to some "inner" activity of the will—a capacity to *choose.* The reason this concept of freedom should be thought of as metaphysical is that no scientific demonstration is capable of proving its existence or nonexistence. The determinist can always claim that a cause does exist, even if we don't yet know what it is. The defender of free will argues that our ordinary concept of choice is both meaningful and applicable in everyday life. Philosophical and theological debates over the shortcomings and merits of the thesis that human beings possess something called "freedom of the will" have raged for centuries. In psychology, positions as far apart as psychoanalytic theory (as first conceptualized by Freud) and the behaviorist views of B. F. Skinner both rest—despite their other differences—on the hypothesis that all human behavior is causally determined. Yet they merely assume rather than prove that people's behavior is determined psychologically. The relevance of the free will–determinism controversy for ethical issues in behavior control is straightforward but complex. The interrelationships go something like this.

Ethics and the Freedom–Determinism Debate

Suppose psychic determinism is true—that all human thought and behavior are caused by events in people's lives beginning as early as infancy, by the genes carrying personality traits, or by some combination of these. How, then, it is often asked, can people be held *responsible* for their actions? If all our behavior is caused, then we cannot be genuinely free agents; rather we would be simply "programmed" to act the way we do. Or, in the language of commonsense psychology, we are "conditioned" to behave in the way we do. This programming or conditioning, in combination with drives or instincts humans share with other animals, is sufficient to rule out anything like genuine freedom of the will. But if we do not have this sort of freedom to choose and act, how can we be held responsible for our behavior? How can we blame those who behave violently, if they cannot help what they do? Why should we punish criminal offenders, if they could not have acted otherwise than they did in committing arson, assault, murder, or rape?

It should be clear that the ongoing debate over free will versus determinism has direct bearing on the treatment of human beings as moral agents. The more likely it is that people have genuine freedom in the "free will" sense, the more appropriate it is to praise, blame, and punish them for their actions. But the more we learn that human behavior is caused by determinants stemming from nature and nurture, the less appropriate it seems to hold people morally responsible for their actions.

Traditional Western religion takes the view that free will is an essential property of persons. The existence of free will is, in this view, a product of God's creation. Backed by religious faith, those who adopt this position see no incompatibility in the view that human beings have free will while everything else follows a deterministic pattern governed by laws of nature. But believers in free will need not derive their position from religious sources. Nonreligious existentialists also believe that this sort of freedom is a basic attribute of human beings. Central to existential philosophy in general, and to its ethical theory in particular, is the view that man is free to choose, that all actions imply implicit, if not explicit, choices the agent makes, and that the attempt to cite causes for human actions is misguided.

The appeal of this view is that it enables us to justify the fact that we do not hold natural forces (such as hurricanes or earthquakes) morally responsible for the destruction they bring about, while we normally do hold human beings morally responsible for their violent or harmful acts. But since this freedom attributed to human beings is basically a metaphysical concept, its presence is impossible to prove by ordinary scientific means. Those who lack the underpinning provided by religious faith must seek some other explanation for how it is that people have this strange sort of freedom, absent in the nonhuman material world.

Scientific psychology, on the other hand, rests on a belief in the determinist ideas about human behavior. Some who adopt this view are prepared to admit that it is impossible to make meaningful moral judgments. If there is no genuine human freedom, then morality is an empty notion. There is no such thing as "human dignity," and we are all equally responsible (or *non*responsible) for our actions. While this position is usually identified with specific theories in psychology, such as the behaviorism of B. F. Skinner, it has long been held as a philosophical thesis independent of any particular psychological position. The apparently bleak consequences for morality have led some philosophers to formulate an intermediate position, one that tries to retain the best of both worlds.

This third intermediate view is sometimes called "soft" determinism, to distinguish it from the "hard" variety that rules out the possibility of freedom and along with it, moral responsibility. The "soft" view is also known as "compatibilism" or "reconciliationism" since it argues that free will and determinism are compatible doctrines; the truth of both positions can be reconciled. The strategy of the compatibilist is usually to show that it is not psychic determinism that is incompatible with human freedom. Rather, it is the notion of *compulsion* that is properly contrasted with freedom. To know whether an act is free, we have only to make sure that certain conditions are not present—that the agent is not "compelled" either by coercive threats of force by other persons or by "inner forces" of uncontrollable fear, rage, or obsession. What should be contrasted with determinism is not freedom, according to this thesis, but rather, *in*determinism—the position that at least some events are uncaused, or random.

This intermediate view has considerable appeal. It allows for the truth of psychic determinism, which seems to be required for a scientific psychology that provides continuity between humans and the rest of the world. At the same time, it accounts for the notion of moral responsibility, which rests on the prior assumption that human beings are free in this sense.

How is the metaphysical notion of freedom, just described, related to the political concept of freedom? The political notion is often couched in terms of individual rights: rights of privacy, of confidentiality, of liberty to behave as one wishes as long as one's actions do not interfere with the same rights of another. The metaphysical concept looks to the inner springs of human behavior. It implies that actions are either uncaused, self-caused, or improperly described as falling within a causal chain of events. These two notions should be kept distinct, since it is possible to promote maximum political liberty for people while still holding that they are not wholly free in the metaphysical sense. Contributing to the confusion is the fact that the term "libertarian" is applied *both* to theorists who believe that people possess genuine free will (the view that psychic determinism is false), and also to those who defend maximum political liberty for the individual against the state.

Coercion and Compulsion

These two senses of freedom, while distinct, are nonetheless related. Both are treated as opposites of the concepts of coercion and compulsion. The political notion of freedom is brought into play in attacks on state control (coercion) of individual behavior. The metaphysical notion of freedom arises in questions about whether people should be held responsible for their actions. The most common grounds for questioning responsibility are that some individuals suffer from a form of psychic compulsion. This consideration arises in some criminal cases, in which the defendant may plead "not guilty by reason of insantiy." Appearing with increasing frequency in recent years are excuses for conduct that point to the fact that victims of prolonged episodes of "brainwashing" could not resist their captors' efforts to remold their values, goals, or motivations. Both notions of freedom bear on the ethics of behavior control in a major area of public policy: both are involved in arguments about what the state is morally permitted to do to its members, and under what circumstances.

Nevertheless, it is common to confuse the notions of coercion and compulsion by treating them as the same concept. For the sake of clarity and to avoid this sort of confusion, the discussions below will use the term "coercion" to refer only to actions performed by one or more persons, aimed at forcing other individuals to do something. So used, it is the opposite of "political freedom." The term "compulsion," the opposite of "free will," will be used to denote inner psychological forces that make some people unable to act other than they do in certain situations.

The nature, kinds, and degrees of psychic compulsion remain a matter of uncertainty and debate among mental health professionals, legal scholars, philosophers, and the general public. Was the seemingly purposeless murder committed decades ago by the pair Leopold and Loeb an act of *compulsion,* as the title of the book based on their actions implies? Was Patricia Hearst truly "brainwashed" and therefore unfree—compelled by her newly and involuntarily acquired beliefs—as psychiatric testimony contended at her trial for bank robbery? While individual cases may remain uncertain, the existence of crippling phobias, as well as disorders such as kleptomania or other obsessive-compulsive conditions, are clear evidence that some people lack the ability to control their own behavior. There is little doubt on the other hand, that the lack of freedom attributed to all human beings by determinists is distinctly different from the inner compulsion suffered by emotionally disturbed individuals who perform acts of theft or violence.

The principle of individual liberty demands maximum personal freedom and minimum state interference socially, politically, and economically. The metaphysical notion of freedom stands at the crossroads of law and psychiatry. Various forms of the insanity defense used in criminal trials rest on the view that the insane should not be held morally or legally responsible for their antisocial acts. There are several different grounds on which a plea of insanity may rest, but the chief assumption underlying all of them is that criminals of this sort lack sufficient capacity to act of their own free will. They are caught in the grip of inner forces of compulsion. In the eyes of the law, culpability must be based on responsibility for actions. Similarly, from the moral point of view, responsibility requires a measure of freedom on the part of the actor. The question of the appropriate treatment of adult offenders who are not "free" to act otherwise than they do remains a central issue of public debate.

Two Philosophical Approaches: Kantianism and Utilitarianism

Debates and uncertainty about the ethics of behavior control often stem from more general conflicts among moral principles or ethical theories. Sometimes ethical theory can be useful in resolving such disputes, but in other cases theory is of no help at all. But even when moral and legal conflicts cannot be settled by this means, it aids our understanding of such disagreements to discover whether the problem lies in the clash of fundamental ethical principles, or in a lack of clarity in the theories themselves. The examination below of two major philosophical theories will serve to illustrate the ways in which their precepts underlie social institutions and public policies.

There are a great many ethical theories in the Western philosophical tradition. Yet two primary channels comprise the mainstream of this tradition. Broadly speaking, one of these channels is the Kantian position, arising from the views of the eighteenth-century German philosopher, Immanuel Kant. The other main current, comprising a wide range of theories, is utilitarianism, whose major spokesmen were the English philosophers, Jeremy Bentham and John Stuart Mill. The utilitarian approach places the feelings, desires, and attitudes of people—especially their pleasure or happiness—at the center of the moral arena. The Kantian notion of morality is focused on the rational being, and rationality is treated as applying to the human species as a whole. The chief trait on which utilitarians base their ethical theory is *sentience,* the capacity for feeling, while the basic human attribute underlying the position of Kant and his followers is *rationality,* the ability to form concepts and to reason. Utilitarians try to ground their ethical theory in a central fact about human beings—the fact of sentience and the accompanying tendency to seek pleasure or happiness and avoid pain. Kantians take an *a priori* approach to the matter of justification, beginning with the concept of rationality and deriving from it the fundamental principle of morality.

Consequentialism and Formalism

The disagreement between Kantians and utilitarians over which human qualities provide the basis for a moral system is not the only feature that distinguishes these two approaches. There is another difference, one that has been the center of considerable philosophical controversy. Just which elements of a situation should be considered morally relevant? Utilitarians take the *consequences* of human actions as the criterion for judging the rightness or wrongness of individual human acts or social practices. The "greatest happiness principle," as formulated by Mill, states that "actions are right in proportion as they tend to promote happiness; wrong as they tend to produce the reverse of happiness. By happiness is intended pleasure and the absence of pain; by unhappiness, pain and the privation of pleasure."[3] Kantians, on the other hand, look to the type or *form* of an action, which is why their approach is often called "formalist." What is important for making correct moral judgments, in their view, is whether or not the behavior "takes the form" of right action, or is the right *kind* of action, To take such form, an action must be done for the sake of duty. Different formalist theories offer different accounts of what our duties are and how we come to know them; some say that right actions are those that conform to certain moral rules. But what all formalist theories have in common philosophically is that they use as the standard of moral rightness the kind of human action performed, not the good or bad outcomes of behavior or social practices.

What binds formalist theories together, then, is that they deny that the consequences of human actions are important for making ethical judgments. The opposite view is precisely what utilitarians and other consequentialists take as necessary and sufficient for making moral judgments. The following two examples of behavior control should serve to illustrate the point.

Illustration: Involuntary Commitment

If someone has committed no crime, yet is judged by psychiatrists to be dangerous to others, the laws of most states provide that the person may be committed to a mental institution. Placing people in a psychiatric hospital against their will is called "involuntary" commitment, to distinguish it from situations in which people voluntarily present themselves for admission to mental institutions. It is also known as civil commitment, to mark it off from incarceration of criminals.

[3]John Stuart Mill, *Utilitarianism,* ed. by Oskar Priest (Indianapolis, Indiana: The Bobbs-Merrill Co., Inc., 1957), p. 10.

Whichever name is used, some defend the practice while others decry it. Those who argue in support of civil commitment laws almost always do so on utilitarian (consequentialist) grounds: To commit such a person has the beneficial effect of preventing harm to others. Whether stated explicitly or not, such moral judgments rest on the probability that better consequences, on the whole, will come about than those likely to result from any other action that could be chosen. Those who favor civil commitment as a social practice seek reasonable grounds for supporting it by appealing to the goodness or badness of the likely outcomes.

In contrast, opponents of involuntary commitment frequently invoke what they consider the overriding value of freedom of the individual. People who have committed no crime or who have violated no law have a right to remain free, this argument goes, and this right carries with it a corresponding duty on the part of others to refrain from interfering with their liberty of action. Those who denounce the practice of civil commitment often appeal to rights and duties of this sort. They reject the arguments that bring in the consequences of refusing to confine persons who may turn out to be dangerous to others.

The resolution of this debate depends not only on agreeing about the priorities of values, but also on the question of facts: How reliable are predictions of violent behavior? This factual matter—the accuracy of psychiatric predictions—is closely linked to the question of which moral principle is the most reasonable to adopt. But even if predictions about the danger to society of particular persons could be made with a high degree of accuracy, disagreement may still remain over the value priorities. This disagreement is likely to stem from an adherence to basically different approaches to ethics on the part of opponents in the dispute. Formalists will not be moved by an argument that appeals to consequences, yet that is precisely what the defender of involuntary commitment often uses to justify the removal of a person's liberty.

Illustration: Punishment

To take a second example—the social institution of punishment—the different justifications offered by utilitarians and formalists rest on a similar set of distinctions. Incarcerating people for crimes they have committed surely interferes with their liberty of action. What should be considered in justifying imprisonment or other forms of punishment for offenders by the state? The standard utilitarian justification is that punishment will deter—the consequences for society as a whole will most likely be good if constraints are placed on any individual offender's liberty. Formalists justify the practice of punishment by invoking the criminal's just deserts.

Deterrent effects are held to operate in three different ways. First, the particular individual who commits a crime is removed from society, so that person is unable to commit additional antisocial acts while incarcerated. Second, it is argued, after being released from prison, the likelihood that a person will commit further crimes in the future is much reduced, because of the fear of having one's liberty removed again. The trouble with this second argument is that recidivism rates among criminals provide evidence that the conclusion is largely false. Being in prison once fails to serve as a deterrent for the large number who become repeated offenders. The third argument is that knowing that imprisonment and other forms of socially mandated punishment exist leads people to commit fewer antisocial and violent acts than they otherwise might. This is a hard claim to prove since virtually every society has used some form of penalty for violation of its norms or laws. Nevertheless, as a justification for removing a person's liberty, the consequentialist argument that punishment has probable deterrent effects stands as a major position.

A wholly different justification for imprisonment is offered by members of the Kantian tradition—the formalists. Known as retributivism, their view holds that criminals deserve to be punished because they have committed wrongful acts. To right the balance of wrongs it is morally necessary to give criminals their just deserts. According to this position, not only does the state have a duty to punish offenders; some retributivists have gone so far as to claim that the criminal has a *right* to be punished. However implausible this view may seem, it has been asserted by as prominent a thinker as the nineteenth century German philosopher Hegel. Arguing along Kantian lines, and against the utilitarian view, Hegel writes:

> . . . Punishment is regarded as containing the criminal's right and hence by being punished he is honoured as a rational being. He does not receive this due of honour unless the concept and measure of his punishment are derived from his own act. Still less does he receive it if he is treated either as a harmful animal who has to be made harmless, or with a view to deterring and reforming him.[4]

Formalists like Kant and Hegel thus reject any appeal to the observed consequences of punishing criminals. The sole legitimate justification lies in the notion that those who have committed a wrong should receive their due according to the scales of justice. This classical version of the retributivist justification has for some years been somewhat out of favor, both politically and among philosophical scholars. Recently, however, interest has reawakened in the "just deserts" model of sentencing and other practices in the criminal justice system. Lawyers and philosophers are now reexamining earlier assumptions and moral justifications in a renewed exploration of the just means of treating offenders.[5]

Both the example of involuntary commitment and that of punishment serve to highlight the crucial difference in approach to moral issues that separates consequentialism from formalism. This does not mean, of course, that philosophers, criminologists, psychiatrists, or most of us in our day-to-day life always act as consistent utilitarians or Kantians in ordinary behavior or in making moral judgments. Nor do moral philosophers choose up sides for one or the other position and then take on the moral issues of the day. Yet those who formulate social policy have available either of two philosophically reputable modes of moral justification: an appeal to rights and duties, or an assessment of the better consequences of having one scheme rather than another.

Illustration: Regulations Governing Research

A somewhat different context for the basic features of both the utilitarian and the Kantian approaches in providing standards for governing acceptable behavior is biomedical and behavioral treatment and research. Therapeutic and research methods for the control of human behavior are a subordinate branch of these, and as noted in the first chapter, problems of informed consent loom large here. The

---

[4]G. W. F. Hegel, *The Philosophy of Right,* in Gertrude Ezorsky (ed.), *Philosophical Perspectives on Punishment* (Albany: State University of New York Press, 1972), pp. 107–8.

[5]For an example, see Andrew von Hirsch, *Doing Justice* (New York: Hill and Wang, 1976).

overall moral standard in current regulations of the Department of Health and Human Services is a blend of the utilitarian and Kantian theoretical approaches. The regulations require that every institution engaged in federally funded biomedical and behavioral research on human subjects have a committee, termed an "institutional review board," whose task it is to review research protocols. In particular, the committee must assess the risk-benefit ratio of proposed research. All new drugs must be tested in this manner, as well as experimental modes of psychosurgery or other physical manipulation of the brain. The institutional review board is supposed to determine whether the benefits of the research will, in all likelihood, outweigh the risks to human subjects. The regulation states that if risk is involved, "the risks to the subject are so outweighed by the sum of the benefit to the subject and the importance of the knowledge to be gained as to warrant a decision to allow the subject to accept these risks."[6] The moral standard embodied in this statement is clearly utilitarian: Even if there is some chance that research subjects will be harmed in the course of the study, the overall benefits (to themselves or others) justify the conduct of the research. The difficulties involved in weighing probable risks of harm against likely benefits, as well as the problems of predicting accurately, are considerable. But on the assumption that it is possible to make such calculations in at least a rough way, the use of risk-benefit equations to evaluate the ethics of biomedical and behavioral research is a good example of a public policy that adopts the utilitarian approach.

Yet the utilitarian standard of morality is not the only one evident in regulations governing biomedical and behavioral research. These same DHHS regulations require that in all instances in which there is any risk to human subjects, their informed consent must be obtained. The informed-consent doctrine, as understood and adhered to in both research and treatment, is not based solely on the ethical principle that people should be protected from undue harm. A strong Kantian strain underlies the practice of requiring a patient's or subject's informed consent—a strain expressed in language such as "the dignity of human beings," "the need to respect personal autonomy," and the individual's "right to decide" what shall be done to his or her person. Federal regulations embody these moral concerns in enumerating several of the basic elements of information necessary to informed consent. Element 1 includes a fair explanation of the procedures to be followed, and their purposes; element 2 mentions a description of any attendant discomforts and risks reasonably to be expected; element 5 cites the offer to answer any inquiries concerning the procedures; and element 6 is an instruction that the person is free to withdraw consent and to discontinue participation in the project or activity. These provisions are aimed at protecting the autonomy of subjects, and in ensuring their freedom to refuse or to withdraw from a study if they wish.

This is thus a mix of utilitarian and Kantian elements in the regulations governing research and informed-consent requirements, but there need be no inconsistency resulting from the combination of the two different moral approaches. The utilitarian balancing of risks and benefits applies to one aspect of research practice, and the Kantian elements in the informed-consent doctrine appear in a different procedure for protecting the rights of research subjects or patients. Often in conflict, these two moral views coexist here without being incompatible as they apply to different aspects of research and treatment.

As long as the debate between Kantians and utilitarians continues to rage

[6] *Code of Federal Regulations,* 45 CFR, rev. as of Jan. 11, 1978.

among philosophers concerned with the foundations of ethics, we cannot reasonably expect a resolution of dilemmas in applied ethics traceable to these different theoretical approaches. But the inability to make a final determination of which theoretical approach is ultimately "right" does not preclude the possibility of making sound moral judgments in practical contexts based on one or the other theoretical perspective. The choice between a utilitarian and a Kantian solution to ethical quandaries is not a choice between one moral and one immoral alternative. Rather, it rests on a commitment to one moral viewpoint instead of another, where both are capable of providing good reasons for acting. Neither is an egoistic or selfish approach, nor is either grounded in privileges of power, wealth, or the authority of technical experts.

Rationality and Behavior Control

The concept of rationality appears in the practical sphere as well as in the theoretical problems that confront the ethics of behavior control. Before turning to the practical concerns, let us take a brief look at the role of this ambiguous yet crucial notion in the context of ethical theory. As mentioned earlier, Kant's moral philosophy assumes that human beings are rational agents. But utilitarian moral theory also has to have some views on rationality. Although the chief human attribute on which utilitarians base their principle is not rationality but sentience, the theory requires moral agents to engage in rational deliberation and calculation. Since acts are right if they tend to produce more happiness or pleasure than any other alternative the agent might choose, anyone who adopts the utilitarian method must be able to think of the available choices, make some assessment of the likelihood of the various consequences, and calculate the outcomes that are most probable and most desirable. To be able to do so, a person must be rational, in a very basic sense.

Conceptions of Rationality

Utilitarian methodology is not limited to decision making in moral contexts, however. A more general approach covers a wide range of personal and policy situations in which people have to make choices and act on them. This approach is sometimes referred to simply as decision theory. Decision theory makes some explicit assumptions about rational choice, in particular, about how individuals should rank the things they prefer. An individual's preferences must be transitive: Anyone who prefers apricots over bananas and bananas over cherries must—in order to be thought of as rational—also prefer apricots over cherries. Preference orderings must also be asymmetrical: someone who would choose an Audi over a BMW cannot—rationally—choose a BMW over an Audi at the same time and in the same respects.

Some further assumptions about rationality are both philosophical and psychological, for example, the view that mature adults are capable of deferring the gratifications of short-range gains or pleasures for the sake of a longer-term goal that is held to be important. This is an aspect of rationality that children usually lack. People acquire it through various life experiences and develop it through maturation.

According to a somewhat narrower philosophical view, rationality is closely linked to the capacity for logical thinking. A person who has a high degree of rationality is good at inductive and deductive reasoning, since these are necessary for being able to select the best means to one's chosen ends. This philosophical conception has a counterpart in cognitive theories in psychology—those that deal with modes of human linguistic and reasoning abilities. Psychological investigations that explore higher cognitive processes study the ability to use language, to think abstractly, and even to engage in lower and higher forms of moral reasoning. All these higher cognitive processes include some aspect of what is generally thought of as rationality. The commonsense conception of rationality distinguishes between acting as a result of careful deliberation and acting from impulse or mere habit.

A somewhat different notion of rationality plays a central role in psychoanalytic theory. According to Freud, the seat of reason is the *ego*, while irrational actions flow from the *id*. More important for our purposes here is Freud's idea that what remains in an individual's unconscious thought processes is irrational, since a person has no access to unconscious thoughts and feelings. People can only behave in a fully rational manner when they are consciously aware of their thoughts, feelings, and purposes. This notion of conscious awareness of one's motives or purposes is a necessary ingredient in the ability to control one's own behavior—to maintain self-control, as discussed earlier. It is also crucial for making the distinction between forms of behavior control that employ the rational processes and those that bypass them.

After looking at some factors involved in making this distinction, we shall explore the question of whether special reasons exist for preferring forms of therapy that employ rather than bypass the rational processes. It may turn out that this is a mere preference—a matter of taste, as opposed to a morally important consideration. Because the concept of rationality is at the center of some philosophical and psychological theories, it is worth exploring reasons for preferring types of behavior-control intervention that use the rational processes over methods that bypass them.

Psychosurgery, the use of psychotropic drugs, and electrode implantation into the brain are prime examples of methods of behavior control that bypass the rational processes. Forms of therapy that work by rewarding ''good'' behavior with things the subject enjoys also fall into this category. An altogether different type of psychotherapy, such as Freudian psychodynamic approaches, or those that appeal to other ''inner'' events—for example, those of Carl Rogers or Albert Ellis, hold that rational processes, in addition to other forces that motivate a person are necessary for a proper understanding, explanation, and evaluation of human behavior. Moral judgments about human actions depend on assessments of the person's rationality, since moral responsibility for behavior depends on the agent's capacity for rational deliberation and choice.

Responsibility for Actions

Some psychiatrists believe that psychopathology is present in every criminal action, and as a result, the perpetrator of a crime should not be held morally responsible (although offenders may be sent to institutions for the criminally insane). If behavior flows from nonrational processes, doesn't this make the agent less than fully responsible in the moral sense? From another determinist view, breaking the law is evidence of an adequate adjustment to a social group that is antisocial, or it may be precipitated by circumstances such as severe poverty or other powerful social forces. Any of these may produce less than fully rational behavior.

Three possibilities exist: All of us share the characteristic that our behavior flows from nonrational sources; none of us do; or only some of us do. At one extreme is the position held by Thomas Szasz and his followers, who are prepared to hold each individual responsible for all his own acts. Existentialists are committed to a similar view.

At the other psychological and epistemological extreme is behaviorism. In this view, no one is genuinely responsible for anything he or she does. The strict behaviorists' brand of psychic determinism leads them to the view that there are no degrees of responsibility. How one behaves is simply a result of schedules of reinforcement. A large number of rewards and punishments are part of our natural background, since we grow up in an environment in which our acts are rewarded by parents, teachers, friends, and others, and it is this history that determines our behavior. Reinforcements may also intentionally or forcibly be imposed on people in hospitals, schools, prisons, or in a therapist's office and are justified by a desire for the improvement, rehabilitation, cure, or overall good of the subject. Moreover, the justification offered sometimes depends on what particular sort of institution a person is in. It may also depend on whether the subject is asked to volunteer or instead—subtly or overtly—is coerced into treatment of some sort, such as behavior-modification programs in prison. This alternative might appropriately be termed "Skinnerian," since whatever its avowed purpose, according to B. F. Skinner himself, behavior modification—like any other technique of behavior control—is "beyond freedom and dignity."

The third position falls somewhere in between the extremes just described. It is represented by various psychodynamic theories in psychology and psychiatry, going back to Plato. In their explanations of human behavior these accounts name such forces as drives, instincts, motives, adaptive mechanisms, reality principles, and human needs. What they all have in common is their ability, derived from their formal structure and the concepts they embody, to distinguish in theory between rational and nonrational processes. In some respects, this view mirrors the age-old, commonsense difference between reason and emotion. Although the distinction here is between reason and compulsion, to the extent that emotion sometimes compels behavior, these categories overlap. Reason may sometimes be the slave of the passions, and then emotion exerts a coercive force over reason. Related, as well, are the views of cognitive-developmental psychologists such as Jean Piaget and his followers (although Piaget largely ignores the emotional aspects of human behavior in his theory). Moral responsibility should be attributed only to agents who have the ability to judge, an ability for which reason is necessary. This still remains the chief trait distinguishing man from beast, according to many psychologists, however they describe the developmental process or the ability to learn in rat, pigeon, or man.

Rational and Nonrational Methods of Behavior Control

Are some forms of behavior control more rational, and therefore more permissible, than others? Are methods that bypass the rational processes less desirable than methods that employ them? Behavior modification is a case in point: Supporters of this method claim that it is among the most *effective* (it works best) and *efficient* (it can be accomplished with least time and effort) ways of changing unwanted behavior.

Critics charge that techniques of positive or negative reinforcement—giving or withholding of rewards—bypass the rational processes. Even if they are more effective and efficient, such techniques may ignore or violate autonomy. Effectiveness and efficiency are values central to utilitarian theory, but they are almost wholly absent from the Kantian approach. A moral standard that emphasizes respect for persons need not take into account the general welfare or overall utility. Especially when utility conflicts with preserving the freedom or autonomy of persons, it is not a morally relevant consideration. Although behavior modification does not rely on technology in the strict sense (compare psychotropic drugs or devices such as intracranial electrodes), it resembles highly technical methods of altering behavior in that it too bypasses the rational processes. Perhaps the term "conditioning" best describes the nonrational aspects involved in the change. Even if behavior modification falls short of the use of full-scale mechanical, electrical, or chemical devices, it is nevertheless a scientifically validated technique for changing behavior—one that claims success and derives from a well-confirmed theory in psychology. Yet to claim that this technique is a nonrational method is not to say that it is used to achieve nonrational ends. People who elect to enter special conditioning programs for, say, agoraphobia choose a rational goal—eliminating a crippling fear.

The main feature of behaviorist learning theory is that learning takes place best—in human beings as well as in animals—by reinforcing or not reinforcing some behaviors, and therefore stamping certain behavior in. Recall that reinforcements are things the organism views as desirable or pleasurable: The desired reward follows certain behavior. An organism does not, strictly speaking, cogitate about whether to engage in future behavior—even though pet lovers might claim otherwise. When used as therapy, behavior modification sets up schedules of reinforcement to change unwanted behavior as originally developed in experimental psychology.

What is nonrational about behavior modification that makes it closer, in this respect, to physical, chemical, and electrical manipulation of the brain than to most "talk" therapies? According to behaviorist theory, an organism engages in a random series of actions toward a goal and as one item of behavior is reinforced, its frequency increases. There is no place in this scheme for free and rational deliberation. If freedom loses its entire meaning, then so, too, does reason: Those two go hand in hand as phenomena that explain human choice and action. Skinnerians are correct to reject both phenomena simultaneously or to accept them simultaneously. But cognitive and psychodynamic schools of psychology hold that it is a mistake to reject both. Convincing arguments show that freedom and reason can be accounted for in a motivational theory of human psychology that acknowledges psychodynamic factors or affirms the existence of higher cognitive processes. Skinnerian accounts have neither of these attributes. Strict versions of behaviorist theory, then, have no place for deliberative mental processes, genuine choice, or reflective rationality.

A theory that does not allow for the distinction between bypassing and using the rational processes is one whose applied methods (whether used for therapy or for social control) cannot make such distinctions either. In some cases, the distinction is rather clear in theory, but becomes blurred in practice. An example is the appeal to nonrational phenomena such as transference (displaced feelings) in psychoanalysis. Yet transference is used in therapy on the supposition that there will always be certain unconscious forces operating in people, since, according to Freudians, we are never totally rational. Destructive unconscious elements need to be understood in the course of therapy so that the person can succeed in changing inappropriate and self-destructive behavioral patterns. Understanding—a rational process—is thus conjoined with the nonrational (emotional) process of transference to bring about a change in behavior. Freud described the results of successful psychoanalysis as rendering the ego—the seat of reason and common sense—free to choose.

Effectiveness and Efficiency

The values on the side of methods that bypass the rational processes, assuming the truth of what psychosurgeons, electrode implanters, psychopharmacologists, and behavior modifiers assert, are those of effectiveness and efficiency. They include the speed or permanence of results, as well as lower financial costs than other methods of behavior change. Behavior modifiers claim to be able to bring about clearly measured changes, in a relatively short time, and in very objective ways. The values on the side of the methods that use the rational processes include the virtue of acting according to reason, adhering to the old Socratic maxim "Know thyself," the subjective feeling of autonomy, and the increased understanding of how to exercise self-control. These values are given prominence even when it is acknowledged that the methods themselves are relatively inefficient.

Some people prefer efficiency, effectiveness, lower costs, and the similar values that accompany the methods by which the rational processes are bypassed. The moral virtue of this position lies in one of its social consequences: Successful psychiatric techniques can be distributed more justly by making them available to more people who need them. This conception of justice is essentially utilitarian, as it rests on the notion that the greatest benefit for the most people is the most just outcome. A preference for values of efficiency and effectiveness over deeper self-knowledge or conscious self-control is a difficult preference to deal with philosophically. It is similar to the kind of clash that occurs in other fundamental moral disputes—as when values like equality and liberty, or individual rights versus social benefits come into conflict. To the extent that efficiency and effectiveness are central values in the utilitarian scheme, the defense of methods that have these characteristics is utilitarian as well.

Ethical issues related to bypassing the rational processes in efforts to control behavior include another significant question—that of responsibility for actions and the ability to justify, as well as to explain, human behavior. Reasons for acting and causes of behavior are not as clearly separable as some philosophers have maintained. Yet this lack of clear separation does not pose problems for the ability to offer reasons for acting, in the sense of "reasons" that justify actions or show them to be rational.

If someone violates the law, the question of whether or not that person was responsible for the action arises: Is he or she competent to stand trial? Does the person "know right from wrong"—The M'Naghten rule in law? Did the individual suffer from an "irresistible impulse"—another legal criterion for insanity? When a person performs morally right actions, and other actions that do not violate the law, should we be concerned that such good behavior was caused by drugs (the sexual offender who no longer goes around molesting little girls because he has been given heavy doses of anti-androgens)? Or by direct brain invasion (for instance, by implanting a miniature electronic device in his brain so that he will no longer steal when he walks into a store)? Or because as a result of understanding and reflection, he has come to see his earlier behavior as wrong and is now sufficiently motivated to change? Are there objective reasons for choosing, developing, further refining, or pouring research money into modes of intervention that use rather than bypass the rational processes? In the search for such reasons, several considerations come to the fore.

One question is whether certain moral considerations override effectiveness and efficiency. In other instances, moral or political considerations outweigh values such as efficiency or effectiveness. Here the answer turns on the factor of potential harm to others. If recidivism rates among criminals are actually lower when methods that bypass the rational processes are used in rehabilitation programs in prisons, this would be a good reason, though perhaps not a conclusive one, for using such methods rather than modes of "insight" therapy. Questions about efficacy of treatment can only by answered by a systematic study of different techniques of behavior control and the results of their use. This is because answering such questions requires empirical evidence, quite apart from any conceptual and ethical analysis that may be necessary.

Additional complications arise from the following consideration. What if a subject (say, a prisoner) is aggressive, with highly charged emotions, yet wants to remain that way? Since control of human behavior may involve changing people's ultimate values or personality structure as well as aspects of their behavior, an inquiry into the moral limits of behavior control must include investigation of the ethical acceptability of altering basic values and personality structures. For the control of human behavior to be morally right, must it be undertaken to meet the subjects' felt needs or interests, according to their own value scheme or expressed preferences? Or is it ethically acceptable for techniques of control to be used by those whose values or preferences for a certain sort of behavior differ from the subjects' own? Would this give the right to alter subjects' basic desires, ultimate goals, or what gives them pleasure in life? The answers to these and related questions depend, in part, on a satisfactory philosophical account of the concept of autonomy. A full theory of the moral limits of behavior control must await the resolution of these prior issues.

A somewhat different factor to consider is the age of the person whose behavior is subject to control. The assumptions that underlie a choice of therapy often rest heavily on particular theories about how and when people acquire the types of behavior they exhibit as adults. According to cognitive-developmental theories in psychology, the attainment of certain abilities and performances at different ages is crucial. But for behaviorists, the question may simply be one of changing unwanted behaviors by a schedule of reinforcement, whatever the age of the person involved. Freudians, too, hold developmental stages to be crucial. It is only an apparent paradox that considerations cited in favor of using behavior modification or other therapies that bypass the rational processes on prisoners are the very things that probably make it worse to use such techniques on schoolchildren, whose minds and characters are still being formed.

What values are in conflict when these different modes of behavior control are under debate? As noted above, efficiency and effectiveness are pitted against the dignity and autonomy of persons. It is obvious that if the very existence of dignity and autonomy is denied, as it is by Skinnerians, no value conflict remains. But you need not be a strict Kantian to acknowledge and seek to promote the dignity and autonomy of the individual. These values are pitted against the presumed benefits to society of efficient and effective modes of behavior change, and it is possible to work toward a compromise between these positions. Seen this way, the issue is not so much what type of behavior control method is used, but rather whether social policies demand respect for the rights of the individual. A balance needs to be struck between honoring these rights and preserving broader benefits to society as a whole.

Reasons for Preferring Rational Methods

Finally, there is the question of what can be considered good reasons for preferring interventions that use rather than bypass the rational processes. One view argues that using the rational processes is intrinsically valuable or inherently worthwhile. This view obviously suffers from all the difficulties of any attempt to demonstrate convincingly that a thing has intrinsic value. Perhaps further support can be gleaned from a position urging that the characteristic of being rational is not only unique to the human species or special in some way, but is also a desirable trait. Rationality is a normative as well as a descriptive concept. In Western culture, rational behavior is almost always viewed positively by the agent, as well as by others. But if this approach rests on the ability to show that there is something intrinsically worthwhile about rational behavior, arguments in support of it will be hard to muster.

A slightly different tack focuses on the instrumental value of being rational. Rationality carries a positive normative force because of its value as *means* to achieving desired *ends*. This part is uncontroversial. But once the premise is added that one of the goals of therapy is to help patients or clients become better able to achieve their ends, then enabling them to use rational processes becomes one of the desired outcomes of therapy. Rationality itself may be hard to defend as an intrinsically worthwhile state or process. Yet it can still have a crucial instrumental value for people in achieving whatever ends they choose. So, if the goal of therapeutic interventions is to produce persons who are, on the whole, more effective in defining and attaining their goals, then the ability to exercise rational processes is one of the desired outcomes of successful therapy. It would be bizarre, at the very least, if the outcome of therapy were described as successful in cases where patients or clients behave less rationally and therefore less effectively, after therapy than they did before. (I leave aside here paradoxical truisms of everyday life, like "it is sometimes rational to act irrationally." Such remarks may make sense after they are explained, but they trade on the multiple meanings of the rich and ambiguous concept of rationality.)

Self-knowledge, insight into the causes or consequences of one's own behavior, an understanding of the motives behind one's actions or failure to act—these seem to be among the central determinants of acting rationally. If these same attributes are also used to characterize therapies that employ rather than bypass the rational processes, then the connection between means and ends becomes somewhat blurred. Rational means used to achieve sought-after ends or desires may themselves take on the character of ends. It is easier to assent to this point than it is to support the stronger claim that the attributes of the ends ought to characterize the means, or the reverse. Rational behavior leads to these characteristic outcomes: the capacity for self-control; an ability to direct one's life purposefully and successfully; and perhaps most importantly, the proper assumption of moral responsibility. These are norms and virtues that people actually strive to attain. In the end, such values may be ones for which no further argument or foundation can be provided. But they remain at the heart of democratic institutions and reflect the importance of the individual in contemporary Western society.

FURTHER READINGS

BENTHAM, JEREMY, *The Principles of Morals and Legislation.* New York: Hafner Publishing Company, 1948.

BEROFSKY, BERNARD, ed., *Free Will and Determinism,* Part One: Alternative Views. New York: Harper & Row, Publishers, Inc, 1966.

ELLIS, ALBERT, *Humanistic Psychotherapy: The Rational-Emotive Approach.* New York: The Julian Press, 1973.

FREUD, SIGMUND, *The Ego and the Id.* New York: W.W. Norton and Company, 1960.

KANT, IMMANUEL, *Fundamental Principles of the Metaphysics of Morals.*

———, *Lectures on Ethics.*

MACKIE, J. L., *Ethics: Inventing Right and Wrong.* New York: Penguin Books, 1977.

TAYLOR, PAUL W., *Principles of Ethics: An Introduction.* Encino and Belmont, California: Dickenson Publishing Company, 1975.

CHAPTER 3

Freedom versus Coercion

A finding of "mental illness" alone cannot justify a State's locking a person up against his will and keeping him infinitely in simple custodial confinement. Assuming that term can be given a reasonably precise context and that the "mentally ill" can be identified with reasonable accuracy, there is still no constitutional basis for confining such persons involuntarily if they are dangerous to no one and can live safely in freedom.

U.S. Supreme Court, *O'Connor* v. *Donaldson*, 422 U.S. 578 (1975)

Mental patients are challenging modern psychiatry, its heavy reliance on treatment with drugs and the whole traditional mental health system.... Mental patients . . . are trying to narrow the controls that psychiatrists have over them in public and private mental hospitals. They want the right to refuse medication and shock therapy, even if they have been committed to an institution involuntarily, and they want more legal safeguards built into the commitment process.... They are also questioning the lexicon of psychiatry, words such as "incompetence," "schizophrenia," and "psychotic." They argue that since psychiatrists frequently disagree on the meaning of these terms, they are of questionable value in commitment proceedings that can mean the deprivation of a person's liberty.

The New York Times, Dec. 11, 1978

The Issues

There is scarcely an American schoolchild who cannot recite the words attributed to the Revolutionary War patriot, Patrick Henry: "Give me liberty or give me death." Although these words were uttered at an earlier time in our society, they express a feeling that is still with us in our moral and political life. Libertarian values are expressed in the slogans of two New England states: New Hampshire's auto license proclaims, "Live free or die"; Vermont's flag warns, "Don't tread on me." With fierce determination, defenders of the value of liberty promote their cause—a cause that requires little defense as a matter of principle, but that comes up against barrier after barrier in practice. Why is liberty such an overarching value, and what are the impediments to its unfettered enjoyment?

It should be clear, first of all, that focusing on ethical issues in behavior control limits our concern to individual liberty or the freedom to act. The freedom of nations from domination by other nations—the target of Patrick Henry's libertarian cry—is not the issue here. The concept of freedom is essentially the same, however, whether it refers to an individual's right not to be coerced by others or to the struggle of one nation to remain independent of domination by another; only the applications differ. Some overlap occurs when the notion of freedom is applied to both individuals and countries. This overlap is best illustrated in a slogan popular in the 1950s and 60s, when debates raged over U.S. nuclear and foreign policy: "Better dead than Red." Embodied in this slogan is the value judgment that death is preferable to an alternative in which it was felt neither this country nor the people who live in it could retain their freedom. The nation as a whole would lose its ability to govern itself if a foreign power were to take over, and the people would lose many individual liberties if the conquering nation were a totalitarian regime notorious for curtailing personal freedom.

Both Patrick Henry's rallying cry and the slogans of recent decades are, of course, bits of political rhetoric, meant to move listeners to action. It remains a matter of speculation whether those who make such pronouncements always take their rhetoric literally. But even if they are not meant literally, slogans that invoke death as the only alternative to the loss of a dearly held value should alert us to the priority such a value may assume in the minds and hearts of those who cherish it. Freedom is perhaps the clearest example of a value often held sovereign over all other values in the moral and political realm.

Freedom as an "Absolute" Value

If freedom really were what it is often called—an "absolute value" (one that should never be overridden, no matter what)—then there would be no moral dilemmas of the sort that crop up when freedom comes into conflict with other values. Nowhere are these dilemmas more starkly apparent than in the area of behavior control. To take the most prominent example: the continuing controversy over the practice of involuntary commitment to mental institutions. Why is this well-entrenched practice so controversial? Precisely because it entails a forcible loss of liberty for people who have committed no criminal act.

People who have violated the law may be imprisoned for the deeds they performed, and only extreme libertarians (usually with an anarchist bent) argue that it is beyond the legitimate bounds of state power to invade an offender's freedom by locking him up. We tend to take for granted the institution of official punishment in society. Whether imprisonment is justified by utilitarians or retributivists, limiting the freedom of criminal offenders seems to be commonly accepted morally. Yet even here we should not overlook the obvious: Incarceration requires making deep inroads into a person's freedom—inroads that would be intolerable if freedom were an "absolute" value. So except for those extreme libertarians who oppose curtailing the freedom of even repeated offenders against the criminal laws, most people would agree that it is justifiable to interfere with individual freedom at least sometimes. The almost universally accepted practice of punishment is enough to show that freedom cannot remain unchallenged as an absolute value. If it did stand over all other values, there could be no justifiable instances of imprisonment, since whenever society jails people who offend against its laws, it places some values over that of personal liberty.

But consider involuntary commitment when no laws have been violated; this is a different story from imprisonment for criminal acts actually performed. The practice of civil commitment is justified in court when the person whose liberty is at stake is judged to be "dangerous to self or others," even when such danger has never been actualized. Why should such judgments, made on the basis of psychiatric testimony, serve as sufficient justification for overriding a value that some have held to be nearly absolute?

According to one school of thought, the answer is simple: There can be no legitimate justification, so involuntary commitment is a moral wrong that should be abolished. In this view, the only proper grounds for removing someone's liberty are those that justify imprisonment, namely, actual performance of a criminal act.

On the opposite side stand two possible views, since justification for taking away someone's freedom depends on the reason offered for involuntary commitment. If someone is judged "dangerous to others," the principle used to justify taking away that person's liberty is the state's duty to protect society from harm. In any but an anarchist political framework, the state is held to have certain obligations to its citizens as well as duties it may exact from them. Just as the state has a duty to defend its populace against harm from without, in the form of threatened invasion by foreign powers, so too does it have an obligation to protect its members from harm by one of their numbers. One who is judged "dangerous to others"—assuming that the judgment is sound—stands a good chance of harming innocent persons, whom the state has an interest in protecting. So interference with the liberty of those who have not (yet) done any harm is held to be warranted on grounds of the high probability that they will commit acts of violence in the future.

The other chief ground for involuntary commitment—"dangerousness to self"—demands a different sort of justification. What business is it of the state's if a person takes his or her own life? Is it a legitimate concern of the government to prevent acts of suicide? It is one thing to seek to prevent harm from befalling innocent persons who may be at risk if a homocidal maniac is on the loose. It is quite another to restrict a person's freedom because he may do harm to himself. If freedom is such an important value, for what reasons can the state remove people's liberty in the most blatant way by locking them up when they have done nothing to harm others and are not even judged dangerous to others? Such reasons can be neatly classed under the heading of *paternalism*.

Paternalism

The meaning of "paternalism" as used here is as follows: "the interference with a person's liberty of action justified by reasons referring exclusively to the welfare, good, happiness, needs, interests or values of the person being coerced."[1] Controlling the behavior of one person is likely to have effects on others as well (family, friends, employers, the community), so actions will rarely be purely paternalistic. Still, we can think of a wide range of uses of behavior-control techniques that are paternalistic in terms of the primary motives of those who employ them or try to justify them.

Why is paternalism such an important moral concept in the domain of behavior control? The main reason is that a wide range of coercive actions and practices rests on a paternalistic grounding. Intervening in suicide attempts and confining people on the grounds that they are "dangerous to self" represent the most extreme cases. Others include sterilizing the mentally retarded and preventing prisoners from volunteering as research subjects. These different practices and policies are all justified by appeal to the welfare, happiness, needs, or interests of members of these groups. It is not the protection of society but rather the individual's own health or well-being that is forcibly assured by paternalistic laws or practices.

Are there any special circumstances in which a person's liberty may be interfered with for his or her own good? What first comes to mind is a situation in which an unknowing person is about to make a false step—over a cliff, into a flame, or onto a banana peel. It may be paternalistic to invade a person's liberty of action by pushing the person out of the way or preventing the misstep in some other manner. But that would be a paternalistic act most people would welcome. The sort people tend to resent—the kind that has given paternalistic acts a bad name—are those in which the person being coerced, instead of being ignorant of some fact related to the deed, seems quite aware of all the circumstances and likely consequences but chooses to go ahead anyway. How, in these cases, can paternalistic acts be justified?

One standard response by those who hold positions of authority or power in medical settings is to identify the subjects of coercion as incompetent. Genuinely incompetent adults are no more capable than infants or children of making sound judgments about their own behavior, this viewpoint urges. Since it is obviously justifiable to interfere in the behavior of infants and small children when they are about to do harm to themselves, similarly it must be permissible to interfere in the behavior of adults who are judged incompetent—the mentally retarded, the senile, or the emotionally disturbed. After all, if they, like children, lack judgment, isn't a certain amount of paternalism warranted?

To ask why some people support paternalism while others argue as forcefully for the priority of individual freedom is to question the psychological causes of moral beliefs rather than the rational reasons for holding them. Many causes, resulting from parental and other influences, determine just which ethical principles any one of us adopts. In the end, we cannot argue about some fundamental princi-

---

[1]This definition is offered by Gerald Dworkin in his article, "Paternalism," *The Monist,* 56 (January 1972), p. 65. Some scholars have argued for different definitions of this concept, but this one is best for our purposes here. A particular virtue of the definition is that it is neutral with respect to connotation. It leaves open the possibility that paternalism can be a good thing, under certain circumstances.

ples beyond a rational limit, but must accept them as basic moral commitments (or as some would say, articles of faith). Those who take one extreme or the other, choosing individual freedom over paternalistic interferences, or the reverse, adhere to this kind of basic value commitment. Intermediate positions are usually easier to defend by good arguments. Yet even in particular cases of disagreement, it may be just as hard to convince someone who thinks it right to coerce others for their own good that paternalism is morally unjustifiable as it is to persuade one devoted to the ultimate value of liberty that an alternative moral position is legitimate. Such impasses are the stuff of which moral dilemmas are made. Yet there is a crucial point to be borne in mind about freedom—a point often overlooked. Sometimes limits placed on liberty of one sort can promote liberty in another area of life. Similarly, some restrictions on liberty in the short run may have the long-term effect of enhancing freedom.

Individual Liberty

Probably the most classic statement of political libertarian philosophy is John Stuart Mill's essay *On Liberty*. Mill, the nineteenth-century British philosopher and social reformer, makes an eloquent statement, rich in detail and broad in scope. Mill's essay is classic, but it is not the most extreme libertarian position. More radical libertarians would not allow the state the authority to set up a police force for the purpose of protecting the people, to conscript men when the nation is at war, to tax earnings—at least beyond a bare minimum—nor to perform many other functions, depending on the details. Taken to its extreme, this libertarian position becomes anarchism; its political opposite is totalitarianism. Behavior control mandated by the state would be, presumably, nonexistent in an anarchist society; on the other hand in a totalitarian regime behavior control exercised by the government over its citizens is likely to be far-reaching. Mill was a libertarian but not an anarchist. He believed in something more than the minimal state, or as it is sometimes called, the "nightwatchman" function of government.

But regardless of where his position falls along the political continuum, Mill's view stands as a major statement, worthy of careful study. The object of Mill's essay, in his words,

> . . . is to assert one very simple principle, as entitled to govern absolutely the dealings of society with the individual in the way of compulsion and control, whether the means used be physical force in the form of legal penalties, or the moral coercion of public opinion. That principle is, that the sole end for which mankind are warranted, individually or collectively, in interfering with the liberty of action of any of their number, is self-protection. That the only purpose for which power can be rightfully exercised over any member of a civilized community, against his will, is to prevent harm to others. His own good, either physical or moral, is not a sufficient warrant. He cannot rightfully be compelled to do or forbear because it will be better for him to do so, because it will make him happier, because, in the opinions of others, to do so would be wise, or even right. These are good reasons for remonstrating with him, or reasoning with him, or persuading him, or entreating him, but not for compelling him, or visiting him with any evil in case he do otherwise. To justify that, the conduct from which it is desired to deter him, must be calculated to produce evil to someone else. The only part of the conduct of any one, for which he is amenable to society, is that which concerns others. In the part which merely concerns himself, his

independence is, of right, absolute. Over himself, over his own body and mind, the individual is sovereign.[2]

Mill holds that it is within the state's legitimate authority to interfere with an individual's freedom of action in order to prevent harm to others. This important condition serves as the basis for a utilitarian justification of the state's rights to punish criminals. Mill's words convey the classic antipaternalist position decrying state intervention into the lives of rational adults. There is little doubt that Mill has in mind people who accurately fit the description "rational adult" when he asserts his principle, as we shall see a bit later.

It is remarkable that the staunchest contemporary defenders of the value of individual liberty—such as Thomas Szasz in the psychiatric sphere, and the American Civil Liberties Union, in the political arena—do not really argue that freedom is the central notion in morality. The ACLU, however, thinks of itself as defending the Constitution, which explicitly guarantees a number of freedoms in the First Amendment. As an activist group, committed to the defense of individual liberty through the law, the American Civil Liberties Union is not expected to provide a philosophical justification for its work in promoting this significant American value. That task is best left to moral philosophers and political theorists.

Unlike many more recent defenders of the doctrine, who lack convincing arguments (if they offer any at all) for their viewpoint, Mill strove to give reasons why it is important to prevent the state from interfering in the lives of its members. The kinds of reasons Mill offered are summarized by a contemporary philosopher:

> *What made the protection of individual liberty so sacred to Mill? In his famous essay he declares that unless men are left to live as they wish "in the path which merely concerns themselves," civilization cannot advance; the truth will not, for lack of a free market in ideas, come to light, there will be no scope for spontaneity, originality, genius, for mental energy, for moral courage. Society will be crushed by the weight of "collective mediocrity." Whatever is rich and diversified will be crushed by the weight of custom, by men's constant tendency to conformity, which breeds only "withered capacities," "pinched and hidebound," "cramped and warped" human beings. . . . " All the errors which a man is likely to commit against advice and warning are far outweighted by the evil of allowing others to constrain him to what they deem is good."*[3]

Mill's claims about what happens when people's liberty is encroached upon might be questioned on factual grounds, and some of the reasons he offers may rest on false psychological assumptions. But he does make a strong case in promoting the libertarian principle. It is important to note that for Mill, the value of liberty is not a matter of individual rights, as it is for other theorists, but rather of general utility. Recall that Mill was a utilitarian, and so was committed to holding that the ultimate justification for any act or practice must lie in its tendency to produce a balance of happiness over unhappiness among all those who stand to be affected. Mill believed that as a matter of fact, maximizing individual freedom contributes to the welfare of the whole.

[2]John Stuart Mill, *On Liberty,* in Max Lerner (ed.), *Essential Works of John Stuart Mill* (New York: Bantam Books, 1961), p. 263.

[3]Isaiah Berlin, "The Notion of 'Negative Freedom,'" in Peter Radcliff (ed.), *Limits of Liberty* (Belmont, California: Wadsworth Publishing Company, 1966), p. 78.

Justifications for Limiting Liberty

Leaving the details of Mill's position for now, let us turn briefly to other circumstances in which limiting people's liberty may be justified, besides those that warrant incarcerating criminals. These circumstances include different instances of protecting society against harm, and also a broader range of cases of preserving the general welfare. All are supported by the utilitarians.

One example mentioned earlier is that of conscripting able-bodied men in time of war. It is surely an extreme constraint on the life of an individual to demand that he give up his job, leave family and friends, submit to rigorous training and rigid discipline, and even risk his life—all for what may be an indefinitely long period of time or a hopeless cause. Yet this is precisely what the military draft in wartime demands. Few people other than genuine pacifists and libertarian anarchists would object to this limitation of liberty when the country has been invaded by a foreign power. For lesser skirmishes and in the case of "unjust" wars there is likely to be much debate about the legitimacy of a military draft. The grounds for debate are largely (but no wholly) factual: Is society really threatened? Are people's safety and property actually at risk? Are the form of government and way of life of the society in real danger? That these are largely factual questions does not automatically make them easy to answer. But how they are answered may have direct bearing on whether intervening in men's lives by drafting them can be justified or not. Facts, as well as values, are thus an integral part of moral reasoning, especially when the approach is utilitarian.

A second instance of interference with people's freedom is the requirement that they be vaccinated when there is danger of an epidemic in the name of public health. While this may not loom large as a form of behavior control, it should not be dismissed as involving no coercion at all. What people are coerced to do may be slight—a one-time visit to a doctor or a center where inoculations are given. But because any medical intervention carries with it some risk, however small, a government requirement that everyone submit to a vaccination—as was long the practice in protecting against smallpox—is a form of coercion, justified by appeal to the utilitarian consequence of better health among the populace. Another public health example of state-enforced compulsion is quarantine or removing to a remote place persons with contagious diseases. Modern wonder drugs and increased medical knowledge and control of diseases such as tuberculosis and leprosy have reduced the need for quarantine and isolation commonly practiced in years past. But the principle remains: If there were an actual Andromeda strain that could wipe out or drastically reduce the population, the protection of society against harm would warrant limiting the freedom of movement of any individuals known to be carriers of the deadly organism.

A third example includes limiting personal freedoms for the sake of justly allocating resources: rationing in time of emergency or under conditions of severe shortage. Government-controlled rationing programs for scarce goods in time of war, bans on watering lawns or limits on water usage during drought, and fixed allocations of fuel are practices that citizens even of "free" societies have come to accept as justified under the circumstances. The basis for such acceptance is the utilitarian calculation that failure to limit the freedom of people to buy or use or do what they want in the short run will lead to almost everyone's being worse off in the long run. An extreme libertarian could consistently hold that limiting freedom in the short run is never justifiable in the interest of long-term goals such as equitable distribution of resources. Yet if the long-term goal is preserving freedom, even an extreme libertarian could remain consistent in accepting state-enforced, short-term limits on liberty in order to maximize liberty in the long run.

The broader we state the conditions that permit inroads into individual freedom, the more we open up areas in which people may be compelled to act according to restrictive patterns. If, instead of "society's protection," we use the words "society's welfare" or "well being" to justify limiting individual freedom, it may license tighter controls on behavior, such as censoring pornography, school busing to achieve egalitarian goals in education, and regulation of the marketplace by the government. It becomes evident that individual freedom is not the only value being served; it has clearly given way to general utilitarian goals.

Competency and Paternalism

The principle of liberty, as urged by Mill and others, appears to prohibit paternalistic interferences with anyone's liberty of action for reasons other than that of protecting innocent people from harm, that is, to promote utility. It seems to rule out intervention into the behavior of suicide attempters, electric shock treatments for mental patients who are opposed to them, and involuntary commitment of those who are judged mentally ill and in need of care, custody, or treatment. Yet to consider the freedom of psychiatric patients to be the only value at stake in psychiatric treatment is too narrow an approach. Other salient values include self-respect, self-esteem, autonomy, preservation of life itself, improving the quality of life, benevolence, humaneness, and justice. Even if arguments in favor of controlling the behavior of rational adults for their own good remain unconvincing, there is still a question about those people who are less than fully competent. We turn next to an examination of this issue.

The word "paternalism" derives its meaning from the notion of treating others in what the dictionary describes as a "fatherly" manner. The clearest paternalistic acts are those of responsible parents or caretakers toward babies and young children. Not only do we think we should interfere with the liberty of action of children in order to protect them from harm, we believe it is our duty to coerce, manipulate, or train small children in many ways. There is usually no quarrel, in principle, with this view. Arguments begin over the particular age at which intervention is no longer justified or about which forms of coercion are allowable, and in what areas of a child's life. But it seems wholly justifiable to constrain the liberty of action of children in their early years, not only to prevent them from destroying themselves, but also to foster their growth and thriving. In fact, it would be immoral to do otherwise.

The clearest cases of unjustifiable paternalistic acts are those in which obviously rational adults, who know what they are doing, are coerced against their wishes, presumably for their own good. This is surely the kind of situation Mill had in mind when he stated his libertarian principle, as a closer look at his position reveals. As the earlier examination of his view showed, Mill would no doubt justify involuntary commitment if a person judged dangerous to others would be likely to commit an act of violence or other harm. On the other hand, he could not readily approve of involuntary commitment on the grounds that someone is "dangerous to self," for that would be paternalistic. But would it be an unjustifiable form of paternalism? Although "paternalism" now usually has a negative connotation, one should avoid thinking of every paternalistic act as wrongful interference, even if one adopts a position that at first appears as strongly anti-paternalistic as Mill's. In applying his principle, we need to ask: Is it always desirable to prohibit interference with another's liberty, or are there exceptions? Mill addresses the question explicitly, but his answer is not wholly clear:

> It is, perhaps, hardly necessary to say that this doctrine is meant to apply only to human beings in the maturity of their faculties. We are not speaking of children, or of young persons below the age which the law may fix as that of manhood or woman-hood. Those who are still in a state to require being taken care of by others, must be protected against their own actions as well as against external injury. For the same reason, we may leave out of consideration those backward states of society in which the race itself may be considered as in its nonage. . . . Despotism is a legitimate form of government in dealing with barbarians, provided the end be their improvement, and the means justified by actually effecting that end. Liberty, as a principle, has no application to any state of things anterior to the time when mankind have become capable of being improved by free and equal discussion.[4]

Even though Mill focused on the laws and actions of government, rather than on the acts or practices of psychiatrists, psychologists, and others who seek to control the behavior of individuals, the issues in both contexts are largely the same. The major task is to produce adequate criteria for judging when individuals are "in a state to require being taken care of by others" or when they are not (yet) "capable of being improved by free and equal discussion." In spite of his stalwart defense of the libertarian principle, Mill might well be prepared to accept a wide range of paternalistic interventions—precisely those directed at human beings who have not attained "the maturity of their faculties." He offers no clear or practically workable criterion for distinguishing between those who have attained such maturity and those who have not; but he nonetheless justifies paternalism for a class of cases. Not only does Mill approve of paternalistic treatment of children—those who are "still in a state to require being taken care of by others"; he actually urges it, as the passage just cited shows. He is quite explicit in holding children and "those back-ward states of society in which race itself may be considered as in its nonage" exempt from his objections to paternalism.

But what about other individuals who are "childlike" in a number of ways, especially in their inability to satisfy the criterion of being able to be "improved by free and equal discussion"? Among these are a majority of those people correctly labeled mentally retarded; many who suffer some form of mental illness, emotional disturbance, or behavior disorder; and the senile. Members of all these groups are not completely rational all the time. Objections to paternalism seem not to apply to people who satisfy Mill's rather vaguely worded conditions—"being in a state to require being taken care of by others" and "incapable of being improved by free and equal discussion." Recall that Mill, in applying his own principle, claims that "despotism is a legitimate mode of government in dealing with barbarians, provided the end be their own improvement." This brand of paternalism is morally and politically repugnant in today's world climate of anticolonialism. Yet it is consistent with Mill's view to believe that it is legitimate to coerce people who are clearly nonrational or incompetent to manage their own affairs, provided the end be their own improvement.

[4]Mill, *On Liberty*, pp. 263–64.

Mill says his doctrine is meant to apply only to human beings who satisfy a second condition: They must be "in the maturity of their faculties." One way to understand this condition is to consider retarded persons, the senile, and those who have what psychiatrists call "thought disorders" not to be in the maturity of their faculties in any but the chronological sense of "maturity." What is meant by "maturity" here is having "fully developed" mental capacities; the lack of full development may be a result of chronological immaturity (children), decline of mental faculties (the senile), disease (mental patients), or unexplained developmental failures (many mentally retarded persons). The law now recognizes an intermediate category termed "diminished capacity"—a category used to mitigate criminal responsibility for some mentally ill or retarded persons who have committed offenses.

Thus, even an attack on paternalistic interference as strong as that which Mill advances allows psychiatrists and others a measure of "justifiable" paternalism in controlling, modifying, or improving the behavior of less than fully rational individuals. For those judged rational (in some appropriate sense of that complex and slippery notion), paternalistic intervention would not be justified.

Rationality and Competence

The problem now is to find appropriate criteria for judging rationality or competence. In this and later chapters the terms "irrational," "insane," and "incompetent" are used interchangeably. This should not imply that these terms have the same meaning, that is, are synonymous. Sorting out the precise meanings and relationships among these notions is complicated, and the chief aim in this book is to explore ethical issues in behavior control and to examine their philosophical underpinnings. Thus less attention will be paid to the wording of various related concepts and more attention devoted to the way they are used in practice, in the law and public policy.

Adults are normally presumed to be rational or competent, and so are allowed to go about their business without interference. Five-year-olds are generally believed to be incompetent in a number of ways relating to their continued health and safety, and so they are watched carefully and their behavior interfered with, when the need arises, by caretaking adults. With the retarded and the mentally ill, it is simply unclear what to assume. We try to avoid erring in either of two opposite directions: being too paternalistic, and therefore unjustifiably coercive, or too permissive, thereby opening the door to their self-destructive or other irresponsible acts. The one evil consists of violating the cherished value of individual freedom (and paternalism may also produce harm if it inhibits proper maturation or development); the other evil is to allow harm, destruction, or even death to befall a hapless, helpless individual.

It is dismaying but not too surprising to discover that the grounds for judging competency are neither wholly objective nor generally agreed upon by experts in the mental health field. There just is no generally accepted, overall theory in psychology or psychiatry on which to base judgments about an individual's rationality, competence, or sanity. Instead, there exist a variety of subtheories and isolated criteria that apply to isolated cases, a small number of which psychiatrists adhere to when they are legally authorized to testify in court. These include very practical criteria such as the ability to test reality and the capability of functioning adequately in everyday life.

In the specific context of obtaining informed consent from the patient or the patient's guardians for treatment, the authors of a recent article in a psychiatric journal describe the various tests of competency used today. They cite as the five basic categories that have been proposed in the literature or that can be readily taken from judicial commentary: (1) evidencing a choice; (2) "reasonable" outcome of choice; (3) choice based on "rational" reasons; (4) ability to understand; and (5) actual understanding. The authors note further that, for a test of competency to be useful, it must be one that can be reliably applied; one that is mutually acceptable to, or at least comprehensible to physicians, lawyers, and judges; and finally, one that is capable of striking an acceptable balance between preserving individual autonomy and providing needed medical care.[5] Thus, while a firm theoretical basis for making judgments of competency may still be lacking, efforts are underway to develop sound practical criteria that psychiatrists can apply objectively.

Yet though a solid theoretical foundation for making legal judgments about competence—judgments that often have direct consequences for licensing behavior control techniques—is lacking, wide areas remain in which people's competence needs to be assessed. One such area consists of legal cases involving the competency of persons to stand trial. A second is that in which criminal responsibility for actions must be determined, and in which the accused pleads "not guilty by reason of insanity." A third is suicide prevention, mentioned earlier in this chapter. Since interference in the suicidal behavior of another person almost always involves coercion, justified by paternalistic reasons, it is worth returning briefly to this topic now.

Suicide and Rationality

Evaluating the rationality of people is a central activity of psychiatrists when they work in cooperation with the law. Debates about the use of coercion on suicidal persons often rely on the concept of rationality. Problems arise from the need to obtain informed consent for recommended treatments, including particular forms of psychosurgery, electroconvulsive therapy, and other procedures. Patients who are deemed incompetent may not—and if evaluated correctly, cannot—grant informed consent when it is required. But this is the very point in question when it comes to suicidal behavior. Is a suicide attempter likely to be judged competent to grant consent, and thus to refuse treatment or confinement? Are suicide attempts rational? Or are they always irrational acts?

According to one prominent psychiatric view, almost all suicide attempts must be seen as irrational acts. In this view important exceptions are suicidal acts committed by the terminally ill, the very old and feeble, or those who feel they are an extreme burden to their family. The view that almost all suicides are irrational is more common among rather more orthodox psychoanalysts. It usually goes along with the moral belief that paternalistic intervention is justifiable as a general rule to prevent suicide. This position has a certain appeal if it is assumed that most suicide

[5]Loren H. Roth, Alan Meisel, and Charles W. Lidz, "Tests of Competency to Consent to Treatment," *American Journal of Psychiatry* 134:3 (March 1977).

attempts are instances of irrational behavior. Paternalism is likely to be morally acceptable when people are incapable—for whatever reason—of using careful reasoning and thoughtful deliberation to make choices or perform deeds. But even if this were true of most people who engage in suicidal behavior, at least at the time of their attempts, it does not follow automatically that involuntary commitment can be morally justified. When it is not known in advance whether the person's behavior is rational or not, is it right to deprive an individual of liberty?

Some who defend paternalism in suicide prevention and control maintain that even if there were sound, generally accepted criteria for assessing rational behavior, it would still be justifiable to intervene in suicide attempts—whether rational or irrational. Defenders of this view often appeal to a duty to preserve life, claiming that this duty overrides whatever duty we may have to refrain from interfering with the liberty of others. Extreme defenders of paternalistic forms of coercion do not need to use arguments of rationality or competence. In the end, the paternalist may not be able to convince the libertarian that involuntary confinement is ever justified. Nor is the libertarian likely to persuade the paternalist. Here, as elsewhere, people hold commitments to different basic moral principles, not all of which are mutually compatible. There is often no rational way of resolving such clashes.

Paternalism: Justifiable or Unjustifiable?

Is paternalism ever justifiable? As usual, when we apply moral reasoning, deciding what is morally the best course of action depends on a mix of conceptual, empirical, and ethical issues. There is surely no easy answer to this question: Under what conditions are acts of coercion, done for paternalistic motives, morally defensible? But despite continuing controversy, a philosophical analysis of the underlying web of concepts, facts, and norms can help to clarify just where the sources of disagreement lie.

It is easy to rebut the claim that all acts of paternalism are morally wrong. In spite of a recent flurry of activity in the "children's rights" movement, few would question the right—or better, the obligation—of parents to interfere in the lives of their preadolescent children, especially when the aim is to prevent some self-destructive act. These are paradigms of justifiable paternalism.

Problems begin as soon as anyone tries to specify the age or conditions when paternalism ceases to be justifiable and becomes, instead, unwarranted interference into the life of a rational or competent person. Those who make the laws have failed to speak with one voice on this issue, so it is of little help to consult judicial opinions or statutes in trying to resolve this moral dilemma. Judgments that it is or is not justifiable to intervene for paternalistic reasons are primarily moral judgments, but they always rest on some underlying factual beliefs as well as on an adherence to a particular conceptual framework. For the purpose of deciding when an individual or a class of persons is sufficiently competent to render paternalistic interference unjustifiable, it is necessary to formulate a small-scale psychological and moral theory linking the notions of competence and paternalism. Parents who consistently apply rules to govern their children's behavior adhere to such a small-scale theory, whether they are aware of it or not.

Conceptual Difficulties

It may be impossible to arrive at a set of necessary and sufficient conditions for applying the concept of competence to a range of people in a variety of circumstances. Thus there may be no way of drawing a sharp line, or one that is hard and fast, in practice. But there is another useful philosophical approach to the problem—the method of paradigms. This method enables us to pick out clear, agreed-upon cases, which gradually shade into gray areas where a concept is hard to apply. There are also truly borderline cases where applying a concept requires a decision rather than a discovery of more facts or theories. Infants and very young children are paradigms of incompetent individuals, if the notion of competency is to have any application at all. This fact, when joined with some common moral precepts and role responsibilities, makes it morally wrong to leave infants and children wholly to their own devices, free from adult care, protection, and intervention. Since the profoundly retarded and the severely depressed have many of the same characteristics as helpless children, the same moral principle applies: Do not let harm befall those who, if left alone, would probably suffer or perish. In the case of parents and children this moral precept is strengthened by the role parents occupy and the special duties and obligations that flow from that role. The borderline cases pose the most difficulty, since the arguments could go either way, depending on how close to the paradigm the analogous cases are drawn. If the notion of being inhumane has any moral force at all, it applies to situations in which those who are clearly psychologically incapable of caring for their own needs are simply left to fend for themselves or perish.

A major problem lies in the fact that disagreement exists over where to draw the line *conceptually* between competence and incompetence. Part of the reason for this disagreement is that competence and incompetence are not discrete, separable states. One shades into the other, and there are different dimensions to consider: People may be highly competent in some respects yet quite incompetent in others. Failure to recognize this can result in mistreatment of those who are classed as incompetent according to specific criteria recognized by the law. For example, those judged incompetent to manage their own finances or to make a will may still be sufficiently rational to grant or to refuse consent for treatment using some medical procedure—say, electroconvulsive therapy. Also, to be incompetent in some ways is not necessarily to be incompetent in all ways. Some mental patients suffer primarily from mood disorders, yet their cognitive capacities remain basically intact. The mildly retarded are slow to grasp concepts and may be incapable of abstract reasoning, yet they may understand, when it is carefully explained, what is involved in sterilization. All this suggests the need for a flexible concept of competence, which would allow for a cluster of criteria to be used when determinations of competency must be made. The result would be appropriately specific judgments of competence rather than the kind of global assessment that is either too sweeping or turns out to be false. In the end, however, disagreement may remain over the question of whether people ought to assume responsibility for others (aside from children, and perhaps their own adult relatives) who cannot care for themselves.

Liberty can only be exercised when a person is in a reasonable state of health (mental or physical) and has reached an adequate age or degree of competence. Unless we hold—as some people do—that liberty is more important than life itself, limitations on freedom are justified in the interest of preserving life or health. Freedom to choose is a hollow value if the individual facing a choice lacks the capacity or the opportunity for rational deliberation, adequate understanding, or reasonable assessment of the consequences of the available options.

The "Best Interest" Doctrine

The discussion to this point has examined paternalistic modes of behavior control and the different factors on which justification depends. But the root conceptual problems connected with the very notion of paternalism remain unexplored. What is the correct interpretation of the notion of ''best interest'' presupposed by paternalism? Is it (1) what those who restrict behavior believe to be in the subjects' best interest? Is it (2) what subjects themselves perceive to be in their own best interest? Or is it (3) what really is in the subjects' interest, where this may be different from (1) and (2), yet can be determined by some scientific or objective means?

Initially, the most plausible candidate for the correct interpretation is (3): what really is in the subjects' interest. The difficulty with this interpretation is that questions of fact shade into questions of value in the area of human behavior. There may simply be no objective way of determining what really is in another person's interest, since that judgment rests as much on preferred values as on discoverable, empirical facts. The problem is compounded by the fact that invasive procedures and forcible means can be used to attain highly desirable ends.

Take, for example, compulsory drug treatment or electrical stimulation of the brain performed on those who engage in acts of self-mutilation; or behavior modification using aversive conditioning on the mentally retarded or on autistic children. These subjects after treatment are often more self-reliant, function more independently, and enjoy a heightened sense of well-being. These qualities are, by general agreement, judged to be desirable or positive ones, and should therefore be considered objective criteria for the purpose of determining what ''really is'' in a person's best interest. In these situations, the subjects' dignity is enhanced; they are enabled to function more autonomously; their self-satisfaction is increased; they are helped to thrive, rather than merely to subsist. These are reasonably clear cases. But what about paternalistically justified modes of behavior control used in prisons and social control of deviants as practiced in mental institutions? Are these actions so obviously for the subjects' own benefit? They are surely practices that those in control, given their commitment to predominant social values and institutional norms, deem to be for the good of those controlled. If the subjects of control disagree about what is in their best interest, their failure to concur may be taken by those in power as evidence that they are less than fully rational and so may justifiably be coerced for their own good.

Even if these conceptual uncertainties were settled, deciding which cases of paternalism are justified and which are not still depends on further facts as well as on underlying values. Consider how a range of facts about the special populations on whom paternalistic regulation is practiced aid in drawing moral conclusions.

The use of powerful behavior control techniques with severely retarded or disturbed persons often promotes their autonomy. Using the same powerful technologies on prisoners may, in contrast, reduce their autonomy, render them more passive and, perhaps, more submissive to the will of others. It is hard to arrive at a fully satisfactory, objective account of which characteristics constitute "changes for the better" as a result of behavior control. In accordance with the Kantian precept that dictates respect for the dignity of human beings, it is a moral requirement for theorists and practitioners of behavior control to promote the independence and autonomy of all persons, even those who are functionally incapacitated or deemed socially undesirable. In the absence of universally agreed upon criteria for determining what really is in the best interests of the subject, paternalistically justified modes of behavior control directed at incompetent persons should always be employed with great caution, but they are nonetheless justified when they are likely to promote autonomy. The question of what are the morally permissible modes and limits of behavior control for the purpose of therapy as opposed to social control will be examined in the next chapter. That topic should not be confused with the subject of the present discussion: What modes and limits of behavior control are morally permissible for paternalistic purposes?

The Mentally Retarded and the Mentally Ill

To conclude this examination of justifiable and unjustifiable paternalism, two special populations about whom conflicting views are often voiced deserve attention: the mentally retarded and the mentally ill. The care and treatment of the mentally retarded has long been the subject of ethical controversy. In earlier decades of this century, sterilization of the retarded was recommended and often practiced for two different reasons. One ground for sterilizing the mentally retarded was that of eugenics: to prevent them from propagating still more retarded persons. The second was primarily for society's protection, based on the belief that retarded persons suffer from a form of degeneracy and that such persons should not be allowed to roam free and endanger the populace. The eminent Justice Oliver Wendell Holmes included both of these reasons in a landmark judicial decision:

> We have seen more than once that the public welfare may call upon its best citizens for their lives. It would be strange if it could not call upon those who already sap the strength of the State for these lesser sacrifices, often not felt to be such by those concerned, in order to prevent our being swamped with incompetence. It is better for all the world, if instead of waiting to execute degenerate offspring for crime, or to let them starve for their imbecility, society can prevent those who are manifestly unfit from continuing their kind. The principle that sustains compulsory vaccination is broad enough to cover cutting the Fallopian tubes.... Three generations of imbeciles are enough.[6]

Both of these beliefs are now held to rest on shaky empirical foundations. The current view is that mild and moderate retardation are forms of developmental disability, transmitted genetically only in a minority of cases. The fears of earlier eras that retarded persons pose a menace to society have also been largely dispelled, partly as a result of increased understanding of retardation, and partly as a result of improvements brought about by better resources. Many statutes allowing for involuntary sterilization of the mentally retarded have been struck down and court

---

[6]O. W. Holmes, Buck v. Bell 274 U.S. 200; 47 S.Ct. 584, 71 L. Ed. 1000 (1927).

cases mandating sterilization overthrown. These legal developments have kept pace with a change in moral perceptions, reflected in recent demands that retarded individuals enjoy all the rights of normal persons, including the right to bear and rear children.

Many advocates of this special population reject paternalistic intervention on the grounds that retarded persons should be allowed to lead lives as close as possible to those of normal persons, even if the process of normalization has some unhappy outcomes for the retarded themselves. Yet some of the efforts of those who educate and care for the mentally retarded include elements of coercion, such as the use of aversive stimuli, with the aim of increasing autonomy and making retarded persons less dependent on others.

When the question of sterilizing the retarded arises, at least the following questions demand careful consideration: Are these individuals competent to grant informed consent for sterilization? If not, is involuntary sterilization ever morally justifiable? If so, on what specific grounds? Is sterilizing retarded persons who would be unable to raise a child an act that is likely to increase or decrease their autonomy? Their overall freedom? Their general well-being? Might sterilization lead to a more normal life in other respects for some retarded persons, even though it blocks their opportunity to bear and raise children? The answer to these and related questions obviously demands an examination of the concepts of autonomy, liberty, and normalization, as well as the empirically necessary conditions for their realization. While it may seem as though sterilization of the retarded or enforced behavior-modification programs are violations of liberty, making their lives less than fully normal, it is important to assess arguments on the other side. Recall an earlier point: Limits placed on liberty of one sort can often promote liberty in another area of life. The mildly and moderately retarded who have been sterilized probably enjoy greater sexual freedom than before, so their opportunity for sexual pleasure can be enhanced at the expense of denying them the opportunity to raise a family. As for young women who suffer more severe forms of retardation, it is frequently in their interest not only to prevent pregnancy but also to eliminate the need for menstrual hygiene. Menstruation itself may be frightening to retarded adolescents. Even the ordinary burdens of personal hygiene are more than many with severe forms of retardation can handle.

The competency of the mentally retarded can actually increase as a result of special education, vocational training, behavior modification, or simply undergoing life's experiences. Nevertheless, their retardation will almost surely remain an enduring trait rather than a temporary condition. So the prospect of paternalistic intervention may continue to arise throughout their lives, since there is little likelihood of their attaining a full state of normalcy.

The situation is somewhat more complicated with the mentally ill, however, since there is greater likelihood that their condition is a temporary one. Consider, for example, a mental patient who has intermittent lapses and remissions and who begs—while lucid—not to have electric shock treatment administered. Is ECT, aimed at improving the patient's condition, justified during lapses when he or she may correctly be held incompetent or irrational? Or should the wishes of such patients be honored on the grounds that their desires were expressed at a time when they were rational agents—persons who deserve not to be treated paternalistically?

Perhaps the hardest cases are those of persons who experience ''manic flights.'' These persons appear rational by virtue of their verbal coherence and occasional bursts of artistic and other creativity. Those who undergo these episodes often refuse even to see a psychiatrist, much less submit to treatment. At least part of the reason is that they enjoy the hypermanic experience.

Why is intervention of any sort felt to be necessary or desirable, and how can coercion be justified? In some instances, those who undergo manic episodes engage in public behavior that threatens their careers, their reputation, their family's well-being, and perhaps even their own self-respect. Sexual exhibitionism, giving away all their money and property, and soliciting 12-year-old boys are typical examples. Realizing the nature of their behavior leads to deep humiliation, at least, and sometimes even to suicide attempts or other self-destructive acts. In many cases, those who are victims of hypermania express overwhelming gratitude—once they have returned to "normalcy"—to psychiatrists, family members and others who had intervened, even over their protests. In all cases, those who exhibit such behavior act uncharacteristically. It is not simply that they act differently from other people—that they are "deviant," in the usual sense. They are deviant in the additional sense that they depart from their own established character. They are not their true selves, they lack continuity with their typical or normal or characteristic personality. Such people appear to be wholly lacking in autonomy when in those states.

To be autonomous in this sense is to have a "self-legislating will," as Kant described it. To be autonomous is to be author of one's own beliefs, desires, and actions. The autonomous agent is one who is self-directed, rather than one who obeys the commands of others. These descriptions of autonomy all presuppose the existence of an authentic self, a self that can be distinguished from the reigning influences of other persons or alien motives. Intuitively plausible as this concept of autonomy seems, it fails to provide workable criteria for distinguishing autonomous from nonautonomous actions in practice. Yet the example of hypermanic behavior is a paradigm—a clear case—of lack of genuine autonomy. How, then, can the autonomy of those who behave out of character, in hypermanic, self-destructive ways, be violated? Autonomous agents, who may sometimes act in ways that others believe are against their own interest, have the right to be let alone. The truly incompetent lack full autonomy, so that quality cannot be violated by imposing treatment. If there is a reasonable likelihood that forced medication will restore or preserve the autonomy of such patients, then paternalism seems warranted by the very precepts that render autonomy valuable in the first place.

In practice, it is rarely easy to determine whether behavior-control interventions are justified for paternalistic purposes. Arguments and evidence on both sides often seem compelling. But whenever such dilemmas arise, they should be tackled systematically by examining the facts of the matter, by keeping clearly in mind the conceptual uncertainty surrounding the notions of freedom, competence, and autonomy, and by exploring the competing values attached to each alternative. A careful, systematic approach will yield solutions that are morally superior to those arrived at by a dogmatic adherence to a stance that either rules out paternalism in principle, or else accepts its legitimacy uncritically.

FURTHER READINGS

BATTIN, MARGARET PABST, Englewood Cliffs, N.J.: Prentice-Hall, Inc.
DWORKIN, GERALD, "Autonomy and Behavior Control," *Hastings Center Report,* 6 (February 1976), 23–28.

LIVERMORE, JOSEPH M., CARL P. MALMQUIST, and PAUL E. MEEHL, "On the Justifications for Civil Commitment," in *Moral Problems in Medicine,* eds. Samuel Gorovitz, Andrew L. Jameton, Ruth Macklin, John M. O'Connor, Eugene V. Perrin, Beverly Page St. Clair, Susan Sherwin, pp. 168–81. Englewood Cliffs, N.J.: Prentice-Hall, Inc., 1976.

SZASZ, THOMAS S., *Law, Liberty and Psychiatry: An Inquiry into the Social Uses of Mental Health Practices.* New York: Macmillan Publishing Co., 1963.

CHAPTER 4

Therapy and Social Control

The freedom of each of us as an individual is restricted by society's interest. The law and morality are expressions of such restrictions. The behavior of a mentally ill person who is not breaking the law is "foolish," "odd," and so on, and society regards it as undesirable.

It is with the protection of citizens from behavior of this kind that psychiatry is concerned. Forcible incarceration in a mental hospital is justified from the social as well as the medical point of view. And if "health" is "desirable behavior" and "sickness" is "undesirable behavior," then the social aim of psychiatry is the transformation of undesirable behavior into desirable. Thus, force used against a mentally ill person is justified by the resulting benefit to society.

A Manual on Psychiatry for Dissidents

... What moral difference does it make if there is a biological impairment? What happens if you just have a kid who behaves in a way that lots of people don't like? And if you find that there's a drug that would cure him, and he and everybody else wants to take the drug even though there is no biological impairment?
... Not cure him. Control his behavior.

"MBD, Drug Research and the Schools,"
Hastings Center Report, Special Supplement, June 1976

The Issues

A man who scales the 110-story World Trade Towers in New York City is nabbed after his successful climb and brought in for psychiatric examination. A daredevil pilot flying his private plane under the low-slung Tappan Zee Bridge that spans the Hudson River is cited for "reckless endangerment" and brought to a psychiatrist. Shocked parents, finding a cache of marijuana in their teen-aged daughter's dresser drawer, decide that their adolescent must be disturbed and seek consultation with a psychiatrist. During disorders on campuses in the 1960s, university administrators and other officials sought help from psychiatrists in their attempt to explain and control violent and even nonviolent behavior of dissident students. Are all these forms of deviant behavior the proper province of psychiatry? Is behavior that departs from what is held to be "normal" automatically a candidate for psychiatric review and diagnosis, and if so, should it be controlled? Whatever the proper province of psychiatry ought to be, this medical specialty has in recent years found its way into broader segments of social behavior with increasing frequency. Over the years a tendency has emerged to label as "sick" a wide range of behavior, from personal and social "maladjustments" such as getting divorced or making a suicide attempt to using alcohol and mind-expanding drugs. This indiscriminate attribution of mental illness has lately come under attack. What are some of the reasons for this attack, and precisely what is at stake?

Major advances in the predictive and technological power of science often bring about striking changes in human activities and institutions. After any significant increase in knowledge or the ability to apply that knowledge, the need arises for new policy stances and review of existing laws that apply to such advances. Much less common are cases in which a scientific taxonomy or classification scheme has ethical, legal, and social impact. Yet a significant example lies in the standard psychiatric diagnostic categories, in which patterns of human behavior and personality types are named and classified. Although these cases are perhaps not as obvious an influence as direct alteration of feelings and behavior through drugs, physical manipulation of the brain, and highly refined behavior-modification techniques, the way in which human behavior is labeled can have far-reaching consequences. Even before effective means of changing mood and conduct were developed, such implications were manifested in the way society treated its deviant members. The history of how people who have been called mad, insane, mentally ill, emotionally disturbed, or "possessed" have been viewed and treated over the centuries is revealing. It is of even more interest, however, when it becomes possible to shape or alter the behavior or personality of society's deviant members instead of simply putting them out of sight or burning them at the stake.

Recent scholarly and popular debate has ranged broadly over these questions, among others: Is mental illness a myth? Are the concepts of mental health and mental illness simply special ways of naming socially approved and disapproved patterns of behavior? Are claims about a person's mental health or illness primarily value judgments rather than scientific assessments? Do the notions of mental health and illness have an irreducible cultural relativity, or is there an objective, cross-cultural basis on which they can be applied?

A second set of issues commanding much attention in the past few years surrounds the problem of "labeling." Labels such as "mentally ill," "retarded," or "underachiever," or those for other socially deviant persons, result in stigmas that often turn out to be unshakable. Such labeling and naming all brands of aberrant behavior "mental illness" overlap, but the problems are not the same. This is partly due to the fact that although the bad effects of attaching a label to someone may last a lifetime, the label itself does not necessarily designate a disease. Children placed in low-achieving groups in grade school may feel, act, and be thought of as stupid—a stigma that may be hard or impossible to shake. But this raises broader issues than the specific problem of labeling *as diseases* some forms of deviant behavior.

The label for a particular form of deviant behavior shapes and influences the way it is thought morally permissible to treat those who manifest such behavior. If a condition is thought of as a disease, there is wide latitude in what it is considered ethically acceptable to submit a patient to in the interest of a cure or in the name of therapy. Invasion of the body, infliction of pain, and even a measure of coercion often seem justifiable when a condition is thought of as a medical one that can be improved by some form of therapy. Treating people in these same ways would likely be viewed with horror, however, if the behavior or condition were conceived of as a product of social choice or merely a "problem in living." Patterns of behavior that cannot otherwise be distinguished from one another are often given widely different treatment morally and legally, depending on just how they are classified in some official diagnostic system.

What are the implications of declaring certain behavior patterns diseases rather than simply forms of social deviance? Does such classification make legitimate certain forms of intervention that would otherwise be illegitimate? Are the results beneficial or harmful to those whose behavior patterns are labeled as forms of illness? Most important, perhaps, are the issues raised by the current technological ability to change behavior and motivation or maybe even to reshape the human personality. It is generally thought not only morally permissible, but even desirable, to change or improve physical deformities or defects in order to conform them to the normal structure and function of the human body. This is partly a medical issue, but it is also largely a matter of values. Can a similar set of facts and values be brought to bear on the question of changing or "improving" personality or behavior? If personality disorders are properly construed as medical diseases, the answer appears to be "yes." The presence of disease is not the sole justification for interventions that aim to change people in the direction of normalcy. Yet a general presumption exists that attempts to "normalize"—where some deficiency exists—are within morally permissible bounds. If people are largely labeled because of their social choice or because of a value classification of the society rather than because of a well-grounded scientific conception of disease or illness, is it ethical to try to transform the behavior or the motivations of such "deviant" persons? Such transformations are often the aim of therapeutic and rehabilitative programs for drug addicts, alcoholics, and many prisoners. There is all the more reason, then, to make sure that programs for behavior change and attempts to alter motivation are entered into voluntarily by those at whom they are directed. As in the use of more invasive techniques, informed, voluntary consent of patients or subjects for behavior-modification treatment is a moral as well as a legal requirement.

The Medical Model and the Concept of Therapy

It might seem easy, at first glance, to make a clear distinction between therapy and social control. The notion of therapy falls squarely within the "medical model"—a way of conceptualizing and classifying people whose behavior deviates in some way from the norm. The use of the medical model has implications, however, that go beyond the theoretical activities of forming concepts and categorizing human behavior and emotional states, calling them diseases instead of lifestyles or ''problems in living.'' There are a number of practical consequences of using the medical model. These consequences bear on how it is proper or even morally acceptable to treat people who are diagnosed as suffering from a disease rather than viewed as exhibiting a preferred lifestyle or experiencing difficulty in communicating with others. But before reaching those consequences, we must first confront the problem of making clear the notion of therapy.

What is therapy? Understood simply, therapy is treatment, the aim of which is to remedy a disease or disorder. Sometimes the remedy succeeds in bringing about a cure for the disease or disorder, as in surgical removal of an inflamed appendix or the use of penicillin to cure strep throat. Other times the remedy only serves to improve a condition that may be incurable, as in the use of L-dopa for persons suffering from Parkinson's disease or chemotherapy to retard the rapid growth and spread of cancerous tissue. In addition, remedies may take the form of palliatives or pain relievers—things that make people feel better—even if the improved feelings stem from the placebo effect. Thus, therapy need not involve remedies that actually succeed in curing an illness or disorder. But the very notion of therapy does seem to involve a treatment chosen to benefit in some way those to whom it is applied. If people are treated in ways that change their physical or mental state without resulting in cure or relief from pain or suffering, whether physical or mental, can the treatment properly be called ''therapeutic''?

Of course, some treatments aimed at remedying a disease or disorder simply fail: They do not succeed in curing or retarding the disease or even in making the patient feel better. But this does not mean that the treatment should not be called therapy in such cases; it does not have to *always* work for a treatment to count as therapy. Whether the failure results from human error or from limitations in knowledge, on the one hand, or instead, stems from the fact that virtually every treatment succeeds only with a certain probability, it is clear that therapeutic efforts do sometimes fail. Yet even when a particular intervention fails, in a given case, if it is similar enough to those that work with some regularity, it may appropriately be considered a form of therapy.

Perhaps it would be more helpful to think of therapy in terms of what it aims to accomplish rather than in terms of its actual benefit to the person. The aim of therapy must be to benefit the individual to whom the treatment is administered, whether by curing the disease, arresting a condition or preventing it from rapidly worsening, or making the patient feel better.

In addition to its aim or purpose, therapy has a second necessary feature: Therapeutic acts must be part of a general practice—an ongoing activity or social institution. Any society has an established and generally accepted body of theory and practice, which provides a rationale for the nature and kinds of actions recognized as therapy. These loose rules governing what counts as therapy may vary from one social group to the next, but every culture has its healers: medicine men, priests, shamans, whether they employ pharmaceuticals, herbs, incantations, or special healing powers. While healing arts and medical science differ from one culture to another, virtually all societies have some practice or practices recognized as legitimate forms of therapy, which can be distinguished from quack remedies, fraudulent practices, and the wholly ineffective treatments that people often seek and demand. Many treatments are widely considered to be therapeutic. But mere belief in the power to heal is not enough for an intervention to be considered a genuine form of therapy.

There are, then, at least two necessary conditions for an action or prolonged activity to be correctly termed therapy. First, it must have the aim or purpose of benefiting the person to whom it is directed; second, it must relate in some way to a generally accepted therapeutic practice. These two essential characteristics of therapy serve to mark it off from two other practices from which it should be kept distinct: activities whose sole or chief aim is social control and those properly viewed as human experimentation. Even if imprisonment turns out to benefit criminals, that does not make it a form of therapy, since the primary aim of imprisonment is social control and not the improvement of the well-being of the prisoner. At least as viewed by utilitarians, imprisonment is justified because it is in society's interest or for the general welfare. When behavior-modification programs are introduced into prisons, it becomes more difficult in practice to draw the line between therapy and social control. Yet the conceptual distinction remains: Both in purpose and in justification, the reason for imprisonment and other forms of punishment is social control, while the primary aim of therapy is to benefit the patient.

For somewhat different reasons, there needs to be a way to distinguish when an action or prolonged activity properly counts as therapy from when it ought to be considered human experimentation. Not only is this necessary to know for the purpose of fully informing those whose consent must be gained for treatment or research activities, but it is also significant for resolving dilemmas about what may ethically be done to prisoners. If castration of sex offenders or psychosurgery performed on those unable to control their violent rages is set in the guise of generally practiced therapy, reactions are likely to be more tolerant than when the procedures are experimental. Leaving aside the problem of whether it is ethical to carry out these highly invasive and irreversible procedures, even if the person has granted fully voluntary, informed consent, we still need to make a distinction between therapy (aimed at helping the subject) and research (aimed at gaining new knowledge). As in the attempt to draw the line between therapy and social control, it is easier to make a conceptual distinction between what is therapeutic and what is experimental than it is to distinguish between them in complex, real-life situations posed by prison settings, mental hospitals, and other social institutions.

Conceptual and Practical Problems

If this account of the notion of therapy is correct, why is there a need to make a distinction between therapy and social control? And why should problems arise in trying to distinguish between them? Let's examine the first question first.

When a condition or form of behavior is labeled a disease, it is natural for people to react negatively to it. In some cases, the labeling may come about as a result of such negative response. Diseases are unwanted conditions, usually (but not always) because those who have them feel badly, are in pain, or suffer loss of functioning. One who complains of disease symptoms is said to have an illness—the experience of undergoing the felt effects of being in a diseased state. It is possible, however, to have a disease yet not to have detectable symptoms; it is also possible for people to have signs of disease but not experience discomfort or loss of functioning. But once diagnosed, diseases are things people strive to rid themselves of, usually as quickly as possible. Sometimes the remarkable self-healing properties of organisms fail to work and the help of outside agents—the skilled hands of a surgeon, powerful chemicals manufactured as drugs, or the sensitive mode of listening and responding called "talk" therapy—is needed. Complications can, of course, arise from even rather simple diseases. And many diseases worsen almost inevitably if left untreated. For all these reasons and perhaps others—such as the human tendency to try to master and control the forces of nature—people dislike being sick and are eager to throw off these unwanted conditions when caught in their grip.

This state of affairs gives rise to several practical consequences of using the medical model for classifying human disorders or statistically deviant conditions. For one thing, once a disorder or form of deviancy is called a disease, it acquires a negative status. It is something to be got rid of, cured, avoided, prevented. Another practical consequence is that diagnosers and healers of diseases acquire a status of privilege and authority, since they are the ones who detect and have the power to cure, improve, or arrest afflictions from which people may suffer and die.

The power held by healers may be subtle or overt. It may take the blatant form that has led to describing what doctors do as "playing God." Or it may exist in the more subtle form conveyed by physicians' own reflections on their efforts to gain fully voluntary, informed consent from their patients. Many doctors confide that they can get their patients to do anything they wish, and that patients often respond to their attempts to gain informed consent with: "I'll do anything you say, Doctor. Of course you know best." Even if physicians do not strive to exercise great dominion over their patients, the nature of the relationship and the healing powers patients ascribe to their doctors give rise to what one psychiatrist calls "the coercive force of the medical model."[1] Although not the kind of force that physicists can measure or for which vectors can be drawn, still it is a force to be reckoned with because of its psychological and social impact. That impact, in turn, helps to show how making the distinction between therapy and social control can have moral implications.

The seemingly neutral acts of conceptualizing and classifying a condition or a piece of behavior as diseased have been shown to possess practical consequences of the sorts mentioned here. Physicians and nonphysicians alike acknowledge that the medical model carries the coercive force that has been attributed to it. As a result, those who take on a therapeutic role are in a position to wield power over those whom they treat. The sufferer from a disease longs to be cured, or at least helped in some way. To that end, the patient may have to undergo assaults that would otherwise be rejected as intolerable. People often endure great pain in the course of many forms of therapy—pain sometimes worse than what they would suffer by remaining untreated. Therapy for burn victims is excruciatingly painful, as are many forms of physical rehabilitation. And many aver that the psychic pain endured for months or even years by patients in psychoanalysis is often worse than the symptoms that led them to seek a psychoanalyst in the first place. Yet in the belief that they have a disease and in the hope that therapy will benefit them, people allow themselves to go through great discomfort and much suffering. It is usually not hard for doctors to convince patients that the cure is worth the painful or disconcerting

---

[1]Dr. Willard Gaylin used this phrase as the title of a lecture delivered at Case Western Reserve University in 1972. A revised version of that talk appears as the Foreword to *Moral Problems in Medicine,* Samuel Gorovitz, Andrew Jameton, Ruth Macklin, John O'Connor, Eugene Perrin, Beverly Page St. Clair, and Susan Sherwin, eds. (Englewood Cliffs, N.J.: Prentice Hall, 1976).

remedy. Not only do people voluntarily undergo unpleasant treatments because of the alleged long-range benefits to themselves, but they are also quite willing, in the name of therapy, to see their infants or children suffer agonizing treatments. Parents would view these same treatments as torture or cruel punishment if administered under some other guise—say, by teachers in elementary school.

Punishment for misbehaving in elementary school is a form of social control. So, of course, is the practice of punishment generally, whether carried out by parents against children or by the state against criminal offenders. The penal system has long been the arm of the law that applies sanctions for violations. Recently, however, medical research and practice have yielded new forms of social control, beyond the traditional ones of incarceration, torture, and slave labor. Ironically, the very same technologies used as forms of therapy in order to benefit people are also employed as means of social control to suppress them. As noted earlier, to be called therapy, an action is to be characterized by its aim rather than by its success in achieving that aim. This is also true of social control: Methods aimed at controlling human behavior so that it conforms to law, to social norms, or to what those in power dictate do not need to succeed in these aims for the label "social control" to be proper. For an action to count as social control, it is sufficient that it be designed to bring people's behavior in line with law, norm, or prescribed conduct.

Some of the most powerful ways of changing human behavior have served both purposes: therapy and social control. Psychosurgery is a clear case. This technique has been used on aggressive criminal offenders and also as a treatment for temporal lobe epilepsy. The same is true of psychoactive drugs and various forms of behavior modification. Virtually any technique used to change behavior can serve the purpose either of therapy or of social control.

Although these two concepts seemed easy to analyze in terms of their meaning and primary purpose, the same clear distinction is difficult to draw empirically. When drugs that act as strong central nervous system depressants are administered to patients in a mental hospital, is the intervention a form of therapy or of social control? As long as patients are diagnosed as having a disease, medication prescribed for that disease naturally falls into the category of therapy. But protests have been raised, alleging that drugs frequently given to patients diagnosed as having common forms of psychosis serve only to subdue the patients, making them more manageable to the hospital staff. While making persons who are out of control more manageable for those who take care of them may be desirable and often necessary, and may be a prerequisite to therapy, it still should not be confused with the activity of therapy itself. Thorazine, a powerful antipsychotic medication that acts as a central nervous system depressant, is one of the common drugs given to institutionalized mental patients. It is worth recalling that this pharmacological wonder was dubbed a "chemical straitjacket" when it first came into use. It is hard to conceive of the original physical straitjacket as a form of therapy. It is, plain and simple, a form of social control masquerading as an odd form of wearing apparel. But just as a straitjacket is neither an item of haute couture nor a treatment that benefits its wearer, so, too, it might be argued, a chemical straitjacket cannot properly be considered a form of therapy if its use serves primarily to render institutionalized persons docile or generally more manageable for the staff.

But it may be too quick to assume that a straitjacket does not benefit its wearer. Precisely the question of whether or not it benefits the wearer is at issue here. The clearest cases in support of the view that physical straitjackets may benefit their wearers are those of self-destructive individuals. In some forms of out-of-control behavior, aggression may be turned in on oneself as readily as outward against others. If restraining a person in a straitjacket succeeds in preventing personal harm that otherwise would not have been inflicted, is the straitjacket not a form of therapy after all, since it does benefit its wearer? The same questions apply to thorazine and other psychoactive drugs, which do not cure or even improve a person's condition unless used continuously. A partial answer to these questions is that not everything that benefits people thereby counts as therapy.

What does it matter what we call it? A straitjacket is a straitjacket, physical, chemical, or otherwise. What difference does it make whether this way of treating people is called therapy or social control? As a first attempt to deal with this question, recall that the law prohibits cruel and unusual punishment of offenders. It also grants prisoners certain rights of privacy and mental autonomy. Our current stage of moral sensitivity leads us to recoil at treatment of prisoners that hampers them by severe physical restraints or employs methods such as immersion in water; most people would be willing to tolerate such procedures in the name of therapy, done in the patient's interest, but not when the purpose is social control.

Illustration: The Hyperactive Child

This point is illuminated further by considering what we believe defensible or permissible in the treatment of children. We balk at the use of corporal punishment in schools, but when physical therapy aimed at improving a crippled child's ability to walk involves exercises causing considerable pain, the suffering is deemed warranted by the expected outcome. In these cases there is no problem in distinguishing between what counts as therapy and what is properly considered social control. A good example of the inability to separate therapy from social control occurs in the practice of administering drugs—in the name of therapy—to hyperactive children in schools. Much controversy surrounds this practice for a number of different reasons.

One factor that fuels the controversy is allegations of ignorance. Medical researchers still know relatively little about the condition called minimal brain dysfunction (MBD), in spite of extensive research over the past several years. In particular, the causes of hyperactivity are unknown; only tentative hypotheses have been advanced. There is also some vagueness about how to mark the boundary separating MBD children (the hyperactive) from the ordinary variety of children (most of those diagnosed as MBD are boys between the ages of six and nine) who are often very active. One difference found through research is that so-called MBD children respond remarkably well to certain psychoactive drugs, somewhat paradoxically, the stimulants amphetamines and Ritalin. Amphetamines, or "speed," and Ritalin have the opposite of a calming effect on most adults. However, in hyperactive children these drugs serve not only to lower their level of physical activity but also to increase their attention span. For children unable to sit still and concentrate, there is little doubt that this medication benefits them in this way. Does this warrant labeling the treatment "therapy?" Opponents of drug treatment for hyperactivity charge the proponents with acting out of relative ignorance.

A different objection raised against the practice of administering amphetamines and Ritalin to hyperactive children—an objection often voiced despite an acknowledgment of the benefits to the children themselves—is based on the setting in which diagnosis and treatment take place. Even if the treatment is properly considered therapy, should it be linked so closely to the schools? Some argue that public schools are not the proper place to administer drugs. They claim that the practice is one more step in the increasing "medicalization" of all sorts of socially deviant behavior. In some cases, hyperactive children who fail to pop their morning pill are sent home from school to take their medicine.

A related objection points out that giving pills to school children as a form of behavior control constitutes just one more "technological fix" in our society. Some hold that there is good reason to shy away from such practices generally, because they tend to mislead the public about the power of technology as well as to promote the search for easy solutions to complex problems. What is worse, in this case, children get the message that popping pills is an acceptable way of affecting mood or behavior, although in another classroom at another time, they are bombarded with anti-drug propaganda under the guise of drug education.

Another line of opposition relies on the distinction between experimental and "accepted" forms of therapy. This objection harks back to the state of medical ignorance both about the causes of hyperactivity and about the nature of the mechanism involved in drug treatment. Because of these unknowns the treatment can, at best, be considered experimental. Some argue that schools are not the proper place for drug research, while others adopt the more forceful line that all drug experimentation on children is risky and should proceed with the utmost caution. The strongest opponents claim that until more is known about the condition for which the drug is prescribed, this treatment ought not be employed at all.

An even stronger line of attack rejects the initial premise of the above arguments—the premise that this treatment is therapy for a disease or medical disorder of some sort. This premise is rejected on the grounds that hyperactivity should be considered a deviant but not a sick form of behavior. If the condition cannot properly be considered a disease, then the therapeutic rationale disappears. Is it, then, right or proper to use drugs on children in school as a form of social control? Many who express this concern are happy to allow parents to take their MBD-labeled youngsters to private physicians for treatment. It's a free society, they claim, and if parents choose to give their children psychoactive drugs under medical supervision, it's their business, but until a clearer medical picture emerges about the nature and causes of the condition currently labeled MBD, drugs should be ruled out as a means of social control in the classroom.

Finally, a prominent viewpoint urges that children should not be labeled hyperactive because of the stigma that accompanies the attachment of any negative label whatever to people. Giving children a label that is likely to stick, or at the very least, will affect their self-image and the way others treat them, is something to be avoided. As long as MBD remains a syndrome about which little is known, it is premature to consider it a disease and to saddle children with a stigmatizing name.

Problems in distinguishing empirically between therapy and social control arise, in part, because the same techniques are used for both purposes. What is more, they may be used in the same settings. In both prisons and mental institutions, for example, behavior modification is used for purposes that can only be viewed as an inextricable mix of therapy and social control. In everyday life an activity often has more than one aim or purpose, and there is surely no reason to think that this same fact of life does not or should not apply as well to controlling people's behavior. The two purposes might not always be clearly separable in the minds of psychiatrists and psychologists, who serve both as agents of social control and as therapists for those who suffer from mental illness or behavior disorders. As a result, it may be impossible to distinguish clearly between their activities in practice.

It seemed easy to distinguish between therapy and social control at the beginning of this discussion by making the purpose of the intervention the central feature. But once it became apparent that a particular intervention may serve multiple purposes, that those practicing behavior control may not be wholly clear themselves what their sole or primary purpose is, and that the same techniques are used for both therapy and social control—often in the same setting—what seemed clear in concept turns out to be not so clear in practice.

The Medical Model Debate

Just as slang terms and expressions in everyday speech go in and out of vogue, so, too, do concepts and ways of referring to items in scientific theory and practice. The notion of a model stems from applications of pure mathematics and logic, but lately the social sciences have adopted model making, and references even in popular literature deal with this way of looking at the world. During the last decade or so the phrase "medical model"—a phrase whose meaning and reference are both ambiguous and vague—has emerged. Since there have been many attacks on the medical model, especially when it encompasses social and political behavior that deviates from the norm, it is important to see clearly the reasons and justification for such attacks. Some contend that the medical or "disease" model ought not be applied to psychiatric disorders such as hysteria or paranoia because ailments having no organic basis should not be conceptualized as diseases, analogous to body ailments. Others argue that it is not so much a question of whether certain forms of deviancy should be thought of as diseases, but rather, of what sorts of treatments are employed and who maintains predominant control over socially deviant persons.

Three Conceptions of the Medical Model

What is meant by the "medical model"? Three different conceptions emerge from writings on this subject. The first of these is a *theoretical* model for the classification and diagnosis of psychological disturbances. In this interpretation of the medical model the terminology of health and illness is used to refer to mental disorders or aberrant behavior of any sort. Those who oppose this variety of the medical model believe that it is a conceptual error to classify behavior disorders as diseases. Disease by definition should be reserved for organic pathological conditions—deviations from the normal biological structure and function of the organism. Those who object to the medical model on these grounds offer a variety of proposals for replacing the well-worn and, in their view, overused medical one. Yet they agree in charging that it is a mistake to conceptualize as illness personal and social behavior merely because it is not well adapted to society's norms, and even if it incapacitates its victims.[2]

These theoretical purists usually have a hidden agenda, however. Their real target is not a mode of classification, but the ethical and social *consequences* of having this particular taxonomy. Among these the most ardent foe of the commonplace idea that there is such a thing as mental illness is probably Thomas Szasz,

[2]Behaviorists generally attack this version of the medical model, as does Thomas Szasz in *The Myth of Mental Illness* (New York: Hoeber-Harper, 1961).

who mounts theoretical arguments against what he claims to be a major error of modern psychiatry. One answer he gives to the question of where this error lies is: "the first error lies in the attempt to elevate the (mental "illness") sufferer, socioethically, from the rank of malingerer to that of patient."[3] By the introduction of such value terms this view goes beyond the theoretical basis for designing a clear, sound classification scheme for all human disorders. Szasz's concern is with the change in human relations that occurs when people are thought of or think of themselves as being ill. The sufferer is to be pitied and is treated as less responsible, more helpless.

These social and ethical considerations form the basis of the second and third common conceptions of the medical model. The second type of medical model is involved not so much with conceptual matters as with *modes of therapy* and the nature of the *therapeutic relationship*. It would beg the question at issue to refer to this relationship as the doctor-patient relationship, since the medical model already creeps in with use of the term "patient." A special quality inheres in the relationship between a healer and the sick person who comes or is brought to the healer for help. While this is generally true of all medical or healing practices, different standards operate in different cultures or even in different segments of the same society. One feature often present in the practice of modern Western medicine is a paternalistic attitude on the part of the medical professional. Along with this stands the authority of the physician. It is this relationship of superior to subordinate, of an expert to one whose consent could never be fully informed, of one in authority who issues "doctor's orders" to the patient layman—this relationship is most typical of the medical model according to the second major conception.

Some who attack the medical model in psychiatry do so in the belief that therapy for the purpose of behavior change ought to be more like a contractual arrangement between equal partners than like the traditional doctor-patient relationship, which is usually between parties in a situation of unequal power. These opponents claim that persons seeking to alter their own behavior should enjoy a more egalitarian relationship with the therapist and have more autonomy than the authoritarian medical model normally permits. Criticism directed at this version of the medical model stems from considerations linked to the theoretical issues embedded in the first conception. The link lies in the reason for rejecting the traditional, medical doctor-patient relationship, namely, the belief that deviant behavior—including neurotic behavior—does not result from some underlying disease of the person. Rather, it is learned behavior, albeit of an unwanted or undesirable kind. There are thus theoretical reasons for questioning some modes of psychiatric therapy, in addition to concerns about the nature of the relationship between therapist and one who comes for help. According to the behaviorist theory that neurotic behavior is learned behavior, if you get rid of the symptom, you have got rid of the disease.[4] If you want to eliminate some unwanted learned behaviors (say, a habit such as fingernail biting), the thing to do is to go to a behavior modifier who will help you unlearn the "bad" behavior and substitute new, "good" behavior instead. What has to be done, according to this theory of behavior disorders, does not warrant a therapeutic approach having features like those of the medical model. Instead, a contractual arrangement is the best means of fulfilling the goal of therapy.

[3] *The Myth of Mental Illness*, p. 26.

[4] This view is expressed in L. P. Ullman and L. Krasner, *Case Studies in Behavior Modification* (New York: Holt, Rinehart and Winston, 1965), p. 2.

The third major conception of the medical model goes beyond the interpersonal matters of the doctor-patient relationship, into even broader ethical, social, and political concerns. In this sense, the phrase "medical model" is used to characterize the predominant medical, social, and legal control over various aspects of mental health institutions and practices in society.[5] Opponents who conceive of the medical model in this sense denounce the role psychiatrists have come to play in the courts. Whether they put the matter as strongly as does Thomas Szasz, who refers to the "conspiracy between law and psychiatry," or simply argue against the use and abuse of the insanity defense in criminal cases, critics are mostly concerned about broad structures of existing psychiatric power. A smaller fraction of those who attack the medical model on broad political grounds sometimes act out of self-interest: Psychologists argue against predominant medical (psychiatric) control over the mental health establishment on the grounds that other mental health professionals should be equal partners on the team.

Most of the time, criticisms are not put forth in one of these pure forms, nor do they raise only one of the concerns cited above. Instead, they are mounted as many-pronged attacks. Controversy surrounding the medical model in recent years has been confused by the ambiguity and vagueness of the very notion of the medical model itself. The result has been that arguments centered on some aspect or version of what is taken to be the medical model are misapplied or unconvincing when directed at others. An understanding of these different conceptions can help us to see more clearly what might be meant by "the coercive force of the medical model." On the second conception, the authority and influence of the doctor often exert a "coercive force" over patient choices and attitudes, even when both doctor and patient think that such decisions are freely and rationally chosen. On the third conception, the role played by psychiatrists in mental and penal institutions, as well as in the courts, amounts to a "coercive force" exercised by a branch of the medical profession over broad segments of society.

Practical Consequences of the Medical Model

If there is no such thing as mental illness, as some opponents of the medical model claim, then it is a mistake to employ medical specialists who allegedly are experts in diseases of the mind, who offer testimony about insanity in court, and who have the power to commit people to mental institutions involuntarily. If there are no mental diseases, how can there be medical specialists whose expertise lies in this field? But even if there do exist some legitimate instances of mental illness, disagreement remains among professionals over just what does or does not belong in this domain. While this may appear to be a mere conceptual or semantic dispute, it has a number of significant practical consequences for law and morality. Given the "coercive force" of the medical model, people who are convinced they have a disease—whether physical or mental—are more likely to seek treatment and be influenced by medical advice. Just as importantly, judges, parole officers, and others in decision-making roles are swayed by medical opinion and testimony. But if a deviant form of behavior is correctly viewed as a lifestyle choice (this view of

[5]This conception is employed by George Albee, "Emerging Concepts of Mental Illness and Models of Treatment: The Psychological Point of View," *American Journal of Psychiatry,* 125:870 (1969).

homosexuality, for instance, is currently supported by many heterosexuals as well as by homosexuals themselves), then it hardly seems as though psychiatric or other medical expertise has anything to offer.

There is a further practical dimension of the medical model, which brings to the fore instructive cross-cultural comparisons. Psychiatric judgments about the behavior of political dissidents can have far-reaching social and political consequences. When political activists are said to be suffering from some form of mental illness or psychiatric disorder—as is the policy of the Soviet Union and, according to some, the United States as well—the way is paved for putting those who disagree with the state's policies or actions into a mental institution. It has been far easier, with the help of expert psychiatric witnesses, to confine political activists and others who display aggressive behavior in a hospital of some sort than to incarcerate those same persons in a penal institution. In addition, it is often harder to gain release from mental hospitals than it is to get a liberal sentence or early parole. So the prospect of abuse of psychiatric power looms large, raising fears that have led some to lay blame at the door of the medical model. A free, democratic society will refuse to sanction locking up people simply because they disagree with government policies. But if dissidents are diagnosed as abnormal, deviant, or sick rather than treated as political activists, the coercive force of the medical model becomes hard to combat.

Deviant Behavior and Psychiatric Disease

Those who claim that there are no such things as diseases of the mind, or that mental illness is a myth, are in a distinct minority. Most American psychiatrists and the educated public acknowledge the existence of mental illness in the form of severe thought disorders, greatly impaired social functioning, and overwhelming mood disturbances. Both psychiatrists and nonpsychiatrists accept or reject a variety of points in between the extremes, along a rather elastic scale that marks off degrees and kinds of psychiatric disease. Thomas Szasz, himself a psychiatrist, rejects even schizophrenia, a classic psychotic condition, calling it and all other alleged mental illnesses "problems in living." The psychoanalytic wing of the profession usually occupies the opposite end of the scale, tending to include failure to engage in "normal" heterosexual relations, problems with authority, inability to find work fulfilling, and poor social adaptations among the ranks of psychiatric disorders.

Critical questions about the medical model and psychiatric disorders are thus practical. Theoretical questions address the appropriateness of construing socially deviant behavior as disease: Is it proper to treat people who fail to adhere to norms and customs as *sick*, rather than simply as odd, defiant, recalcitrant, or rebellious? Is the implication that such individuals are *unable* to conform, or just *unwilling?* Should a pattern of behavior properly be considered a disease if the actor experiences little or no sense of distress? Does it make a difference for the appropriateness of classification if a biological basis for the deviant behavior is discovered?

If it does make a difference, it is important to see why. It is probably true that both our conception of persons and the notion of normalcy contain implicit reference to a biological state that can be considered optimal. More is known about physiological and biochemical contributions to human health and well-being than about corresponding psychological factors. Also, since some form of discomfort or suffering usually accompanies disease, critics have been led to deny that a number of personality disorders—where feelings of distress are often absent—should count as disease. If organic abnormalities and feelings of distress are both missing, what grounds remain for judging those who engage in aberrant behavior as "sick"?

Practical questions include worries about the high degree of subjectivity that is an inevitable feature of the judgments psychiatrists make when diagnosing deviant behavior patterns. How much in degree and kind does an individual have to deviate from particular social norms in order to be judged as having a psychiatric disorder? Are psychiatric judgments likely to be biased depending on the strength of the clinician's own approval or disapproval of the nonconforming behavior?

Other practical considerations link more directly with the distinction between therapy and social control: Are those who fail to conform to society's norms or the prevailing cultural milieu made better off or worse off by being classified as sick? What sorts of behavior-control interventions are warranted when deviant behavior is seen not as sick, but instead as antisocial or criminal?

Responsibility for Actions

If there is one central notion that lies at the core of this knot of problems, it is the concept of responsibility for actions. When people are considered not responsible for what they do, it does not make sense to make moral judgments about their behavior. It does not make sense partly because of the way moral concepts function in our language: A requirement for their correct use is that the actor being judged is acting freely—he could have done otherwise. When people cannot hold themselves back from doing something; when they are caught in the grip of an inner compulsion or are pushed or tugged or shoved by outside physical forces, they cannot be considered free to act otherwise. This is the sense meant here by acting freely—the absence of compulsion, from without or within.

There is another reason why it does not make sense to pass moral judgments on the actions of people who are not responsible for what they do. The first reason was conceptual; the second is pragmatic. It is only part of the role of moral judgments to describe or report behavior. Another chief function is to guide actions. The very act of uttering a moral judgment usually has some effect on the actor whose behavior is being praised or blamed. And there may be even further effects to follow, in the form of punishment, reward, or other sanctions imposed on the one who did the deed. All these activities occurring in the moral arena rest on an underlying premise: Praise or blame, punishment or reward, can have some effect on the future behavior of the one to whom they are applied. No amount of moral prompting or punishment can alter the behavior of people who cannot do otherwise than they do in their choices and actions.

Here, then, are two convincing reasons why it does not make sense to pronounce moral judgment on the behavior of those who cannot be held responsible for their actions. If it would be wrong to praise or blame people who cannot help what they do, so, too, would it be wrong to punish them. To call a thief a kleptomaniac is to acknowledge that he steals out of compulsion, that he therefore has an illness, and so cannot respond to punishment. To inflict punishment on someone whose behavior will not change as a result, and who was not responsible for certain acts in the first place, because of illness, smacks of vengeful cruelty. Responsibility for actions, then, is the key moral concept underlying social sanctions and penal institutions.

If someone's behavior exhibits noticeable changes—perhaps the person is more irritable, perhaps he even goes into violent rages—first reactions might be to assume him responsible and to lay blame. If it is later discovered that this man has a brain tumor and that the tumor is causing his out-of-control behavior, immediately he is no longer held responsible. In an instant he becomes a patient, no longer a moral agent. When a brain tumor is identified as the culprit, it absolves the person from moral responsibility for his actions. Here again, some consequences of adopting the medical model are evident. Suppose that everything in the foregoing situation is the same except that no tumor or brain lesion is found. No sign of physical pathology emerges after a thorough medical work-up and extensive tests. To call a behavioral disorder a disease, whether physical or mental, serves to absolve the afflicted one from responsibility for his actions. What holds for pressure on the brain from a tumor should apply as well to psychic pressure that compels actions. People caught in the grip of inner compulsions, whether their outlet takes the form of rage, theft, or senseless, repetitive acts, are not acting freely. If they are called sick, what they are perceived as needing is therapy, not punishment.

This is the rationale behind having two sorts of institutions to house criminal offenders. One type of institution—the prison—is where those who are held responsible for their criminal acts are incarcerated. The other type of institution—the mental hospital—is for those who may have committed identical acts but are not held responsible. But it makes sense to have two different sorts of institutions for criminal offenders—one penal, the other therapeutic—only if there is a difference in their function, treatment personnel, or methods of behavior control. We shall return to this issue in the next chapter when institutions and alternatives are examined.

There is, then, a seeming oddity in a system that treats certain behavior as at once criminal and sick. Construed as diseases, psychiatric disorders should excuse their victims from criminal acts performed as a result of the illness. So long as it is possible that the same type of deed—let us say, rape—may be either a manifestation of a personality disorder or, alternatively, simply a freely chosen act of sexual violence, it is not terribly puzzling that one and the same type of behavior may be viewed as at once criminal and sick. Some rapists would then be judged to be sick, while others would be deemed evil. This assumes, of course, that there are independent criteria for judging the rapist to be suffering from a psychiatric disorder. If the act of rape itself serves as the criterion for attributing a disease to the sexual aggressor, there is no way, in principle, for a man to commit rape and not be suffering from a personality disorder.

Where disease and criminality overlap, as they do in a number of psychiatric disorders, use of the medical model is confusing, but often introduces humane factors into how offenders are treated. Where do criminals diagnosed as suffering from a personality disorder belong? In prisons or in mental hospitals? If they are victims of disease, it is not only folly to punish them; it is blatantly immoral, for they cannot help what they do. If drug dependence and drug abuse are psychiatric disorders, it is inappropriate and perhaps inconsistent to hold addicts criminally responsible for use and possession of narcotics. The notion of rehabilitation, as employed in the penal system, offers a convenient way of continuing to blur the distinction between therapy and social control. Rehabilitation has some of the elements embodied in the notion of cure: It implies setting a situation right, bringing people back to "normal." But it glosses over the crucial concern of responsibility for one's actions.

Social and Political Impact: Two Cases

Two striking cases highlight the ambiguities inherent in treating aberrant behavior as a disease of some sort. The first is drawn from American psychiatry, the second from Soviet psychiatry. In the American example, the practice of homosexuality, formerly classified as a disease in the official diagnostic scheme, has now been "de-listed." In the Soviet example, the behavior of political dissidents is classified as a form of schizophrenia. Both of these situations illustrate how social and political factors may be closely intertwined with theoretical and clinical matters in behavior control.

Homosexuality No Longer a Disease

Until 1973, homosexuality was officially classified as a personality disorder, included in the category of sexual deviation along with transvestism, pedophilia, fetishism, and sexual sadism (including rape, sexual assaults, and mutilation). The American Psychiatric Association diagnostic manual referred to all of these as "pathological behavior," so there is little doubt within the profession about their official status as a disease. Over a period of years, under pressure from homosexual groups and in response to changing social attitudes, the American Psychiatric Association altered its official position on the classification of homosexuality. While some homosexuals suffer distress as a result of their condition and have sought the help of psychiatrists in trying to change their sexual orientation, others affirm total satisfaction with their sexual preference and insist that they are making a lifestyle choice in remaining homosexual. At the annual meeting of the American Psychiatric Association in May 1973, a high-ranking official of the organization urged its members to stop labeling homosexuality as a mental illness. He charged that this policy amounts to a misuse of psychiatry and results in detrimental social and legal consequences to homosexuals. This statement met with varied responses. One psychiatrist agreed with the view that homosexuality should not be categorized as a disease, but went on to cite studies carried on since 1962, which "leave us with no doubt that homosexuality is not normal. . . . The notion that it is, is a myth promulgated largely by the militant homosexual organizations."[6]

In December 1973, the board of trustees of the APA voted to abandon the position on homosexuality it had held for almost a century. They did agree to categorize some instances of homosexuality as instances of "sexual orientation disturbance," dropping the term "mental disorder." But the category of "sexual orientation disturbance" was intended to include only those individuals who are disturbed by their sexual orientation and wish to change it. The trustees added: "This diagnostic category is distinguished from homosexuality, which by itself does not necessarily constitute a psychiatric disorder." In the same meeting, the board of trustees passed a resolution deploring discrimination against homosexuals in housing, employment, and licensing. The then president of the organization noted that whether homosexuality should be classed as a sexual deviation had been the topic of a growing debate, "fanned by the organized homosexual community, which has vigorously protested the prejudice that derives from classifying their condition as a mental illness."

---

[6]This quotation and the accompanying details were drawn from news reports in *The New York Times* dated May 10, 1973, and April 9, 1974, and the *Washington Post,* April 9, 1974.

Finally, about four months later, a referendum on the matter was held among the APA membership. The vote was demanded by the members after heated debates followed the action by the board of trustees—an action opposed by many psychiatrists. The APA leaders acknowledged that their decision was strongly influenced both by changing social attitudes and by pressure from homosexual organizations. One psychiatrist observed: "It is indeed saddening to see the American Psychiatric Association functioning more as a church council deciding matters of dogma and philosophical speculation than as a professional scientific organization."

Among the confusions that need sorting out here, one of the most pressing is an answer to the question "what is normal"? In the debate about homosexuality, some psychiatrists are adamant in asserting that the condition is not normal; others take the side of members of the homosexual community who deny that it is abnormal. A psychiatrist from Columbia University's College of Physicians and Surgeons claimed: "We're not saying that homosexuality is either 'normal' or 'abnormal.' We're saying that homosexuality per se is not a psychiatric disorder." How should these assertions be properly understood?

Most of the confusion stems from systematic ambiguities in the concept of normality. The term "normal" can refer either to a statistical frequency or to a notion of normative correctness—a value concept. On the first meaning, to show that an action or behavioral pattern is normal is simply a matter of determining the frequency of its occurrence. There may still be quibbles about just where to place the cutoff point: Does behavior have to occur with a statistical frequency higher than 50 percent in order to be considered normal? Or should divorce now be considered normal, in this statistical sense, because one out of two marriages ends in divorce? Quibbles aside, the meaning of "normal" in the statistical frequency sense should be clear.

On the second meaning, the claim that an action or behavior pattern is normal expresses a value judgment. To say that divorce is abnormal, in this sense, is to make a statement about what is right or proper, what ought to be the case. It should be obvious that an act can be considered normal in one of these senses and abnormal in the other. The way Nazi SS officers treated Jewish prisoners may well have been normal in the statistical sense, but few besides other Nazis would declare it normal in the normative or evaluative sense. When these observations are applied to homosexuality, it is easy to see how confusions arise in interpreting the concept of normality. When homosexuals and their advocates assert that the condition is not abnormal, they are appealing to the normative sense of the concept. Their message is: Do not pass value judgments on homosexual conduct. But this is fully compatible with the truth that homosexual patterns of behavior are in the distinct minority statistically. Those who argue that homosexuality is not abnormal would be making a silly factual error if "normal" referred only to statistical frequency. But debates about whether or not some statistically infrequent behavior is nevertheless normal are not (for the most part) silly arguments, although they are often confused.

The psychiatrist who denied that the APA was saying that homosexuality is either normal or abnormal was seeking to make a further distinction. When he claimed that the APA was saying that homosexuality per se is not a psychiatric disorder, he was making a point about the scientific taxonomy: Whether homosexuality is normal or abnormal in the statistical sense, and whatever value judgments anyone might make about this sexual orientation, it is a conceptual mistake to consider it a disease. To see that this view is plausible, we need only observe that not all disapproved patterns of behavior are diseases: Having dirty hair or fingernails is not a disease, nor is breaking promises or treating others rudely. Neither are all statistically deviant conditions diseases: Having an IQ of 180 is not a disease, nor is the ability to run the four-minute mile.

Sorting out confusions about the concept of normality does not, however, succeed in resolving other sorts of problems with the American Psychiatric Association's decision to remove homosexuality from the ranks of personality disorders. Recall the remarks of the psychiatrist who likened the APA's action to a church council deciding matters of dogma and philosophical speculation. His concern was whether the factors that led to the decision emerged from scientific considerations or altered theoretical conceptions within psychiatry, or rather, stemmed from social and political forces. The debate among psychiatrists—the experts in the field—did not address matters of psychological theory, but focused almost wholly on the social and ethical impact such a change in classification would have on the lives of homosexuals. Whatever the theoretical soundness of calling homosexuality a disease or a nondisease, the decision to change the official classification went forward. Practically speaking, it matters not whether the moving force was political pressure from gay activists or moral concern on the part of psychiatrists for the social plight of homosexuals. What the sequence of events suggests is that disease labels applied to or withdrawn from modes of deviant behavior can be as much a matter of social choice or political expediency as they are an outcome of psychiatric theory or clinical practice.

Political Dissidence as a Disease

The "coercive" force of the medical model is nowhere demonstrated more clearly than in the blatant abuse of psychiatry in the Soviet Union. The labeling of many political dissidents as insane, their incarceration and harsh treatment at the hands of medical personnel, and their difficulty in obtaining release are elements in a situation that has worsened over the past decade and a half. Instead of rounding up those who criticize state policy in speech or in writing and treating them like political prisoners, as in former times, Soviet authorities more recently have chosen to call native spokesmen for freedom and justice "schizophrenic." Those who charge that the relationship between psychiatry and the law in the United States amounts to a conspiracy would do well to reflect on the literal truth of this indictment as applied to the situation in the Soviet Union.

Hospitals have traditionally been viewed as a more humane alternative for society's deviant members than prisons, both because of the difference in personnel and in the way inmates are treated. Yet the treatment of political inmates in special hospitals in the Soviet Union is judged by some, who have experienced both, to be worse than that in jails or labor camps. One form of "treatment" consists in the administration of potent drugs such as Haldol (described in Chapter 1), which help the sick but have frightening neurological effects on normal people. To make matters worse, those treated are often denied counteracting medication, which would provide some relief from the awful side effects of these powerful drugs. Unlike ordinary criminal proceedings under Soviet law, those who are accused of crimes, and as a result dubbed mentally ill, are committed to a mental hospital, where they lose all legal rights. Once committed, political prisoners alleged to be insane can remain confined for an indefinite period of time.

Soviet psychiatry offers a graphic instance of the way insidious forms of social control can be achieved under a guise of therapy. The words of two Soviet political dissidents, Vladimir Bukovsky, a human rights activist, and Semyon Gluzman, a protesting psychiatrist, convey a clear picture of the ethical, legal, and social dimensions of the current situation. Bukovsky and Gluzman met in the Perm labor camp in 1974 and together wrote *A Manual on Psychiatry for Dissidents*, which was secretly smuggled out and published in the West. In the Introduction to this manual, Bukovsky and Gluzman write:

> *It is well known that in the Soviet Union today large numbers of dissenters are being declared insane, and there is reason to fear that this method will be used on an even greater scale in the future. It is not difficult to find an explanation for this phenomenon. From the point of view of the authorities, it is an extremely convenient method; it enables them to deprive a man of his freedom for an unlimited length of time, keep him in strict isolation, and use psycho-pharmacological means of "re-educating" him; it hinders the campaign for open legal proceedings and for the release of such people since even the most impartial man will, if he is not personally acquainted with a patient of this sort, always feel a twinge of uncertainty about his mental health; it deprives its victim of what few rights he would enjoy as a prisoner, and it provides an opportunity to discredit the ideas and actions of dissenters and so on.* [7]

What are the features of political dissidents' behavior that enable psychiatrists to make convincing judgments about their insanity? Essentially two diagnostic labels are used by Soviet psychiatry in its interpretation of dissent from government policy as a form of insanity. One of these labels is "sluggish schizophrenia," the other "paranoid development of the personality." A textbook for students at medical institutes includes the following symptoms of "sluggish schizophrenia": unsociability, sluggishness, loss of interest in life, mild attacks of pessimism and melancholia, concentration on inner experiences, inadequate thoughts and actions, stubbornness and inflexibility of convictions, and suspiciousness. The term "sluggish" refers to a form of the disease in which these symptoms are barely apparent, while overt symptoms such as hallucinations are not present at all. This loose definition of schizophrenia is a product of the "Moscow school of psychiatry," which for a time stood in contrast to the rival "Leningrad School," adhering to a more rigorous definition.

Among the features picked out by the other chief diagnostic label, "paranoid development of the personality," two types of "delusional states" are significant:

> *(a) Reformist delusions: an improvement in social conditions can be achieved only through the revision of people's attitudes, in accordance with the individual's own ideas for the transformation of reality.*
> *(b) Litigation mania: a conviction, which does not have any basis in fact, that the individual's own rights as a human are being violated and flouted; the reasons become "clear" to him, and he begins to send in complaints and demands to have "justice" restored.* [8]

There is no better way to discredit a person's beliefs, statements, and actions than to pronounce him mentally ill. Labels such as "schizophrenia" and

[7]Vladimir Bukovsky and Semyon Gluzman, *A Manual on Psychiatry for Dissidents*, 1974, p. 1. Reprinted and distributed by the U.S. Committee Against the Misuse of Psychiatry, Washington, D.C.

[8]*A Manual on Psychiatry for Dissidents*, pp. 7–8.

"paranoia" carry over a strong sense from their conventional use in psychiatry, where they are names for incapacitating psychotic disorders. So the impact of giving outspoken critics of the government a label that ordinarily denotes a severe thought disorder cannot be overemphasized. It is one of the most effective ways of discrediting past actions and maintaining ongoing control over those of whom the state disapproves. Some comparisons between the situation in Soviet psychiatry and elements of forensic psychiatry as practiced in the United States may be apt. But it remains instructive to witness the differences, in the moral and political realm, between behavior control in a totalitarian regime and behavior control in a free society.

The distinctions made in this chapter between therapy and social control, and between deviant behavior and psychiatric disease, will recur when we consider the treatment of criminal offenders in the next chapter. Two considerations crucial for ethics emerge from these distinctions: treatment programs for criminal offenders, where the "right to refuse treatment" has become a major concern; and the use of the insanity defense in criminal trials. Let us turn now to a range of issues surrounding institutions and the available alternatives that exist within them, as well as some alternatives to the practice of institutionalization itself.

FURTHER READINGS

DWORKIN, GERALD, "Can Convicts Consent to Castration?" *Hastings Center Report* 5 (October 1975), 17–18.

HALLECK, SEYMOUR L., *The Politics of Therapy*. New York: Harper & Row, Publishers, Inc., 1971.

KITTRIE, NICHOLAS N., *The Right to be Different: Deviance and Enforced Therapy*. Baltimore: Johns Hopkins Press, 1971.

KLERMAN, GERALD, "Can Convicts Consent to Castration?" *Hastings Center Report* 5 (October 1975), 18–19.

ROBITSCHER, JONAS, *The Powers of Psychiatry*. Boston: Houghton Mifflin Co., 1980.

SCHRAG, PETER, and DIANE DIVOKY, *The Myth of the Hyperactive Child and Other Means of Child Control*. New York: Pantheon Books, 1975.

SIEGLER, MIRIAM, and HUMPHREY OSMOND, *Models of Madness, Models of Medicine*. New York: Harper & Row, Publishers, Inc., 1976.

SZASZ, THOMAS S., *Ideology and Insanity*. New York: Doubleday and Co., 1970.

WENDER, PAUL H., *The Hyperactive Child*. New York: Crown Publishers, 1973.

CHAPTER 5

Institutions and
Alternatives

—We have separated the bad from the mad. We have held the "bad" responsible for their actions and, therefore, subject to judgment by the criminal justice system. The mad we have said need treatment. . . . For both categories of deviance, the bad and the mad, we have attempted to create institutions that would simultaneously provide incarceration and treatment. We have wanted to satisfy the needs of both constituencies—those of the society at large that has demanded retribution and restriction of the physical movement of deviants, and those of the deviant for rehabilitation.

GERALD L. KLERMAN, M.D.
The Hastings Center Report, August 1975

—But what kind of crusade is it to condemn sick and fearful people to shift for themselves in an often hostile world; to drag out, all too commonly, a hungry and derelict existence in a broken-down hotel if they are lucky; victimized, if they are not, by greedy operators of so-called halfway houses that are sad travesties on a fine concept? All without their even knowing the possibilities of new medical approaches to their illness—and all in the name of "civil liberty."

New York Times Editorial
Apr. 8, 1975

The Issues

This chapter is about alternatives. Alternatives of several different types pose moral dilemmas for society's effort to control the behavior of some of its members. As we have seen in earlier chapters, there exist a variety of psychological and technological methods, each having one or more justifications for its use. What binds together the alternatives discussed in this chapter is their relationship to institutions whose purpose is to house individuals society deems in need of custody. As Gerald Klerman observes in the quotation above, rehabilitative and retributive models both operate in the type of living arrangements known as "total institutions."

Common usage of this phrase to refer to a variety of settings sharing common characteristics arises primarily out of the writings of the sociologist Erving Goffman. In his book *Asylums* Goffman writes:

> When we review the different institutions in our Western society, we find some that are encompassing to a degree discontinuously greater than the ones next in line. Their encompassing or total character is symbolized by the barrier to social intercourse with the outside and to departure that is often built right into the physical plant, such as locked doors, high walls, barbed wire, cliffs, water, forests, or moors. These establishments I am calling total institutions. . . .[1]

Characteristics of the type Goffman lists do not enable us to distinguish between the two major types of total institutions in our society—prisons and mental hospitals. Sociological characteristics describe what is, but rarely embody what ought to be, as judged according to normative criteria. To inquire into ethical issues in any domain, it is often useful and almost always necessary to know a range of relevant empirical facts. But the process of moral decision making requires a move beyond the facts. The most common step is to add value premises of some sort to an argument. In moral reasoning, the justifications on which arguments rest have both factual and ethical premises. A defense of the practice of placing society's deviant members in total institutions must appeal to some such value premises. So, too must the attempt to introduce alternatives to institutionalization.

Psychiatrists and psychologists have been greatly influential in administering and giving direction to alternative types of programs for both prisoners and mental patients. Yet these mental health professionals do not usually find themselves in situations where they are asked to give a moral justification for their accepted practices or ongoing rehabilitative programs. Once the requirement to justify acts and practices in total institutions is faced, alternatives begin to present themselves. As we saw earlier, justifications for imprisonment sometimes rest on a retributivist foundation and at other times are based on values drawn from utilitarian theory—deterrence, rehabilitation, or other considerations intended to maximize the general welfare. We also examined the reasons for involuntarily committing those who have performed no criminal act. The justification for committing persons judged "dangerous to self" or "in need of care or treatment" is necessarily paternalistic. But when the grounds for commitment are not paternalistic, a different set of moral problems emerges. For those judged "dangerous to others," the chief difficulty lies in making accurate predictions of the probability that they will perpetrate harmful acts. Some psychiatrists have argued that their discipline offers little guidance to

[1]Erving Goffman, *Asylums* (Garden City, N.Y.: Anchor Books, 1969), p. 4.

practitioners who are called on to make such judgments in court. The search for alternatives demands close attention to the current state of knowledge in the field of mental health. It also requires a careful sorting out of the different moral justifications for confining people in institutions.

Two major facilities exist in our society for housing "undesirables." This chapter will examine different sorts of alternatives these institutions and their justifications pose, as those alternatives relate to behavior control. The next section will look at the grounds that legally justify placing deviant individuals who have committed the same type of act in one or the other of these institutions. As an alternative to criminal incarceration, the insanity defense enables lawyers to enter a plea on behalf of their clients of "not guilty by reason of insanity." These defendants have been charged with committing a crime, often with good evidence in support of the charges. If successful, an insanity plea renders the offender not culpable in the eyes of the law. Whether law-breakers are sentenced to jail or, alternatively, sent to a mental hospital for the criminally insane, is a choice that should properly be based on the perceived sanity or rationality of the offender, assuming that such determinations can be made.

In addition to the insanity defense, two major issues call for investigation: alternatives *within* institutions and alternatives *to* institutionalization, as the latter have come into vogue since the beginning of the "deinstitutionalization" movement in the 1950s and 60s. These "inside" and "outside" alternatives overlap in a number of ways that will become clear as the analysis proceeds.

The optimism with which the attempt to remove chronic inmates from total institutions was originally greeted has waned considerably as the ethical and social tradeoffs have become evident. Even more disappointing to many psychiatrists and criminologists has been the falling out of favor of the rehabilitative model—the dominant ideology over the past few decades in prisons and mental health facilities. The programs designed for inmates in these institutions, as well as the justifications for them, had been based on the optimistic goals of cure and reform, rather than the earlier notions of punishment and retribution. Those who seek humane alternatives to mere incarceration continue to look for ways to avoid the degrading and often hopeless atmosphere of the total institution. These efforts sometimes draw on advances in behavior control technology and at other times proceed by devising new social arrangements.

Both imprisonment and commitment to a mental institution intrude deeply into the lives of those who suffer this fate. It is no less an intrusion even when the legal dictates of due process are carried out to the last minute detail. Incarcerating criminals in mental hospitals rather than prisons has generally been thought of as the more humane of the two alternatives; yet in the last several decades, a wide range of abuses in mental as well as penal institutions has been uncovered. Public sentiments have also changed, with the result that judicial decisions have mandated the "right to treatment" for those institutionalized as emotionally ill or as mentally retarded. The recognition that involuntary confinement in a mental institution constitutes an unacceptable infringement of individual liberty eventually led to a number of landmark judicial decisions (*Rouse* v. *Cameron; Wyatt* v. *Stickney; Donaldson* v. *O'Connor*).[2] These cases focused primarily on the right to treatment, but also

---

[2]Rouse v. Cameron, 373 F.2d 451 (D.C. Cir. 1966).
Wyatt v. Stickney, 344 F. Supp. 383 (M.D. Ala. 1972).
Donaldson v. O'Connor, 493 F.2d 507 (5th Cir. 1974).

included a number of subsidiary rights guaranteed to incarcerated persons. The court's opinion in *Wyatt* v. *Stickney* listed the following rights, among others: the right to the least restrictive conditions necessary for treatment, the right to be free from isolation, a right not to be subjected to experimental research without consent, the right to a comfortable bed and privacy, the right to an individualized treatment plan with a projected timetable for meeting specific goals, and the right to adequate meals.

Value Tradeoffs

Alternatives of various sorts have been suggested for criminals, as well as for the mentally retarded and the emotionally disturbed. The chief question posed by the presence of alternatives to incarceration is as follows: What are the moral gains and losses that arise from institutionalizing offenders rather than using other modes of managing or monitoring their behavior? Two examples will illustrate the dimensions of the ethical dilemma.

As an alternative to spending the remainder of their lives serving a sentence of life imprisonment, two convicted child molesters requested that they be castrated—a procedure medically termed "bilateral orchidectomy." A San Diego judge approved these requests in early 1975. Both defendants were forty-five years old and had prior histories of sex offenses involving minors. Such operations had formerly been common practice under judicial orders in California, but for a number of years preceding this case surgical castration had generally been opposed by the courts since the American Civil Liberties Union brought suit against a San Diego judge and a surgeon involved in a similar operation.

Faced with the likelihood of being confined to prison for a lifetime, the two men signed requests for surgical castration, along with waivers releasing their lawyers, the surgeon who was to perform the operation, and the judge who approved the request. The judge delayed sentencing the defendants, claiming that the surgery would constitute "part of a rehabilitation program which might contribute to a possible grant of probation."[3] In the meantime, the surgeon spoke with medical colleagues, all of whom advised him against doing the operations because of the legal risks. The physician noted that "these men may have voluntarily sought the operations and signed waivers, but is it really a free world decision on their part when their only alternative is probably life imprisonment? Is that duress? Certainly they cannot be said to have made a judgment under the best mental conditions." Several months later the defendants were sent to prison for indefinite terms following an unsuccessful quest for a surgeon willing to perform the operation. Referring to one of the prisoners, the judge lamented: "A whole branch of the medical profession has been unwilling to extend a humanitarian service to this man, who faces the prospect of being locked in a cage for the rest of his years." A compelling feature of this dilemma is the very nature of the value tradeoff: Is it ethically acceptable for society to grant criminal offenders the option of a form of self-mutilation in exchange for their freedom, when one of the purposes of the state is supposed to be to *protect* its members from harm?

A second example of a value tradeoff serves as a reminder that modern

---

[3]Details of this case and quotations attributed to the judge and the surgeon were drawn from news reports in *The New York Times* dated May 6, 1975, and October 2, 1975.

technology offers more alternatives in the realm of behavior control than ever before in history. The authors of a book entitled *Psychotechnology: Electronic Control of Mind and Behavior,* report on prototype testing of a remote radio-communications system using belt transceivers. They describe the device as follows:

> Systems of this type can monitor geographical location and psychophysiological variables, as well as permit two-way coded communication with people in their natural social environment. Probable subjects include individuals susceptible to emergency medical conditions that occasionally preclude calling for help, (e.g., epilepsy, diabetes, myocardial infarctions), geriatric or psychiatric outpatients, and parolees. It is conceivable, for instance, that convicts might be given the option of incarceration or parole with mandatory electronic surveillance. In terms of cost . . . , treatment effectiveness, and invasion of privacy (few situations are less private than prison), an electronic parole system is potentially a feasible alternative. These systems can also be used for positive secondary reinforcement of prosocial behavior.[4]

The authors, who openly favor the development and use of these forms of psychotechnology, correctly point out that one form of privacy (or its invasion) would be traded for another if such devices were offered as alternatives to incarceration. But there is not only an exchange of different types of privacy here; the loss of privacy for the parolee is offset by a corresponding gain in freedom to move about in society. Freedom and the right to privacy are two highly prized values that usually go hand in hand in Western culture. The problem of having to choose between them is, therefore, especially acute and not so easily resolved as these writers seem to think.

With these examples serving as a backdrop against which to examine institutions and alternatives, the following questions summarize the key issues:

In the choice between alternatives to or within institutions, what values are at stake?

Are moral principles in conflict? If so, what are they?

What is to be gained or lost, in any particular case, by implementing alternatives to or within institutions?

What empirical facts or scientific theories are necessary for resolving an ethical problem about alternatives, and in what way are they relevant?

How should social policy regarding behavior control be formulated, in light of this set of facts and values?

Who ought to be involved in making actual policy decisions that offer behavior-control alternatives: The inmates themselves? Administrators (often psychiatrists) in charge of institutions? Committees consisting of psychiatrists, lawyers, representatives of the public (whoever they be)—or even philosophers?

Moral Ideals and Social Policy

Five moral concerns or ideals are central to ethical and legal debates and should be incorporated in social policy. First are all the concerns related to personal

---

[4]Robert L. Schwitzgebel, "Emotions and Machines: A Commentary on the Context and Strategy of Psychotechnology," in Robert L. Schwitzgebel and Ralph K. Schwitzgebel, eds., *Psychotechnology: Electronic Control of Mind and Behavior* (New York: Holt, Rinehart and Winston, 1973), p. 15.

liberty, often referred to politically as the "rights of the individual." These have been pressed in the form of legal demands or moral requirements defending the right of self-determination in matters affecting the life, physical and mental health, and general well-being of inmates of total institutions.

Second, there is the conceptually separate but practically related notion of autonomy. As we have seen earlier, this concept refers to the psychological determinants of people's decisions and also to the values they independently arrive at or the practices they engage in reflectively, rather than out of habit or as a result of being coerced. Ethical issues concerning institutions and alternatives often involve—explicitly or implicitly—an appeal to the value of people retaining or regaining their autonomy, in this sense of the term.

A third consideration in weighing behavior control alternatives is the question of whether paternalistic intervention can be justified when it is clear that the individual is likely to suffer from self-destructive or harmful behavior. This may result from self-neglect, stemming perhaps from drunkenness, depression, or depravity.

A fourth moral notion, also covered in previous chapters, is the legitimate function of the state in protecting innocent members of society from harm. In those states where the legal grounds for involuntary commitment are couched in terms of "dangerousness to others," the value of allowing those so judged complete liberty is held second in priority to the idea that the government ought to provide for society's protection.

Finally, a weaker version of the moral principle just cited shades into an aesthetic consideration. Some members of society strongly desire the removal of grossly deviant people from public view. There is, admittedly, a fine line between what those who wish to "sanitize the streets" think of as morally repulsive or offensive to decent standards of public behavior, and what counts as genuine harms. Are there any objective standards based on psychological or psychiatric theory? Doubts about this possibility were explored in the last chapter. Still, there is an important difference between acts like murder, mugging, and mayhem, and the behavior of sexual exhibitionists or those who drool and talk to themselves loudly in public. My own view is that arguments resting on the social importance of sanitizing the streets by removing deviants are grounded largely in aesthetic values rather than those more properly seen as moral considerations. Yet they do become inflammatory issues when proposals are advanced for deinstitutionalizing mental hospitals or setting up community homes for the retarded. The release to public life of those locked in protective environments offends some and strikes fear into others, whether or not fear or offense are reasonable or warranted. Fear of radically deviant individuals, usually born of ignorance of their condition and tendencies, adds a psychological dimension to these considerations. Where objections to deinstitutionalizing deviant but nondangerous persons rests on fears stemming from uncertain expectations, the issue is no longer just an aesthetic one.

An analysis of these multiple moral factors and how they should bear on social policies must ultimately take into account empirical facts both about life within institutions and also what consequences result when inmates are released from (or never committed to) asylums for the bad or the mad or the incompetent. But as many social scientists and even a greater number of philosophers have at long last acknowledged, hard facts and empirical evidence are rarely "value-free," especially in social settings. It is worth recalling that even when the best data are available, the facts never "speak for themselves."

The Insanity Plea:
An Alternative to Criminal Responsibility

The law has long recognized an excuse that can absolve criminals from guilt for their actions. The prevailing form the insanity defense has taken since the middle of the nineteenth century, dating from the M'Naghten Rules in England and a few years later the United States, allows an alternative to holding offenders responsible for their criminal acts. This alternative has enabled people to be acquitted of crimes in an increasing variety of circumstances. To cite only three examples in recent years: a New York City policeman, having shot and killed a fifteen-year-old boy, claimed temporary insanity on grounds that he had had an "epileptic psychomotor seizure," which caused him to hallucinate a (nonexistent) gun in the hand of the youth he subsequently shot. The jury accepted this defense and ordered the police officer committed to a state hospital. In the second example, a woman stabbed her husband to death in their home, though not in response to his violence or aggression at the time, claiming in her defense that he had beaten her frequently and that she killed him to protect herself. A hearing was held to determine the woman's fitness to stand trial for homicide; she was judged insane and committed. In a third case, a woman poured gasoline on her former husband's bed and set it afire, killing him. In her defense she claimed that he had moved back into her home after they were divorced, and once again begun to beat her as he had when they were married. This woman, too, was acquitted on the grounds that her deliberate arson was an act of temporary insanity.[5] These verdicts, absolving a person of criminal responsibility, decree that persons who have committed such acts are not guilty by reason of insanity. Originally introduced as a humane measure, the insanity defense in law has come under fire over the past few decades.

There are three main reasons for undertaking an examination of the insanity defense in this chapter. First of all, an inquiry into the philosophical rationale for separating the bad from the mad would be incomplete if it failed to address this subject. An examination of the underlying reasons for making this distinction, as well as the criteria employed by courts, continues threads begun in earlier chapters where rationality, competency, and responsibility for actions were discussed.

A second reason flows from considerations explored in the last chapter. When the insanity defense is used in legal proceedings it is necessary to have "expert" witnesses testify to the criminal's insanity. These experts are usually psychiatrists, although in some jurisdictions psychologists have gained similar authority. We have seen sufficient reason to question some basic assumptions behind the idea of psychiatric expertise. Psychiatrists often disagree among themselves, offering alternative general explanatory theories as well as different hypotheses regarding the mental condition of particular individuals. Also noted earlier were some doubts about the very concept of mental illness—today's preferred way of referring to the condition still legally termed "insanity." There remains a distinct lack of theoretical agreement on the meaning or even the meaningfulness of the terms "mental illness" and "insanity." If it is hard to agree upon a genuine subject matter about which one can be expert, then the idea of granting mental health professionals the privileged position of giving "expert" testimony in court is both theoretically unsound and morally in error.

[5]These cases and a number of others are discussed by Hugo Adam Bedau in "Rough Justice: The Limits of Novel Defenses," *Hastings Center Report* 8 (December 1973), pp. 8–11.

The third main reason for discussing the insanity plea here is that it illustrates clearly the power and authority psychiatrists have acquired in established legal practices and in a variety of institutions for the control of behavior. (The final chapter discusses the political dynamics of this situation in greater detail.) Changing interpretations of the insanity defense and the introduction of new legal rules with increasing frequency are more often the products of shifting trends in law and changing political currents than they are a reflection of advances in psychiatric theory or practical wisdom. Nevertheless, psychiatrists continue to play a central role in the judicial process.

The power to offer testimony that may result in a determination of what type of institution a criminal is to be committed to is one that ought not be abused. If psychiatrists do lack genuine expertise in distinguishing the bad from the mad, yet occupy a status that confers the authority to make judgments that determine an offender's fate, abuses that are both unwitting and unnoticed may well take place. Scientific, moral, and political concerns become entangled and confusing in the welter of debates over the use, abuse, and possible abolition of the insanity defense as an alternative to a plea of "guilty" in the criminal law.

Legal Rules Used in the Insanity Defense

Lack of theoretical agreement on the meaning and correct application of the terms "mental illness" and "insanity" has resulted in the continued acceptance and use of unscientific criteria for assessing criminal liability. The leading example of this is found in the century-old M'Naghten Rules. The heart of this doctrine is as follows:

> ... *every man is presumed to be sane, and to possess a sufficient degree of reason to be responsible for his crimes, until the contrary be proved ... ; and that to establish a defence on the ground of insanity it must be clearly proved that, at the time of committing the act, the accused was laboring under such a defect of reason, from disease of the mind, as not to know the nature and quality of the act he was doing, or, if he did know it, that he did not know he was doing what was wrong. (The Rules in M'Naghten's case (1843), 10 Cl. and F.200 at p. 209.)*

In addition to more general criticisms leveled at the insanity defense, the M'Naghten Rules have been charged with a special defect:

> *From the start English critics denounced these rules because their effect is to excuse from criminal responsibility only those whose mental abnormality resulted in lack of knowledge: in the eyes of these critics this amounted to a dogmatic refusal to acknowledge the fact that a man might know what he was doing and that it was wrong or illegal and yet because of his normal mental state might lack the capacity to control his action. This lack of capacity, the critics urged, must be the fundamental point in any intelligible doctrine of responsibility.*[6]

According to this charge, the M'Naghten Rules are defective because they provide only a cognitive criterion for judging the absence of full rationality or sanity. A cognitive criterion, couched solely in terms of belief or knowledge, is too narrow to succeed in sorting out rational or sane from insane persons when the purpose is to determine responsibility for *behavior*.

[6]H. L. A. Hart, *Punishment and Responsibility* (New York: Oxford University Press, 1968), p. 189.

The M'Naghten Rules have been replaced or supplemented in many jurisdictions by a second criterion—the so-called rule of "irresistible impulse." Also used to obtain a defendant's acquittal on ground of insanity, this rule absolves the agent of legal responsibility "if, by reason of the duress of . . . mental disease, he had so far lost the *power to choose* between the right and wrong, and to avoid doing the act in question, as that his free agency was at the time destroyed." (*Parsons* v. *State,* 2 So. 854, 866-67, Ala. 1887.) This criterion for determining the absence of criminal responsibility focuses not on any defect in the agent's thinking or reasoning but rather on what is called a "volitional" defect: the inability to translate into action what one (cognitively) believes to be morally right or socially appropriate. The "irresistible impulse" rule thus rests on a different psychological basis than the M'Naghten Rules.

"Control tests," as the irresistible impulse rule is sometimes called, appear to suffer from difficulties of their own. Consider the following passage from the Colorado law, which represents one version of the modified M'Naghten Rules:

> . . . *care should be taken not to confuse such mental disease or defect with moral obliquity, mental depravity, or passion growing out of anger, revenge, hatred, or other motives, and kindred evil conditions, for when the act is induced by any of these causes the person is accountable to the law (Colorado Revised Statutes 16, 8, 101; 1973).*

It is surely questionable whether "expert" witnesses or laymen who serve on juries can make these theoretical discriminations or find out enough in practice about the defendant to warrant trust in their ability to keep distinct what they must take care not to confuse.

Another major legal test of insanity was the Durham Rule (*Durham* v. *U.S.,* 214, F2d. 862, 1954), abandoned only eighteen years after it was introduced. It stated that "an accused is not criminally responsible if his unlawful act was the product of mental disease or defect." The rule was criticized on grounds of vagueness in the expression "the product of mental disease." In addition, lawyers attacked the rule on grounds that questioned psychiatrists' ability to say when an act is *not* a product of mental disease, even if they are capable of telling when an act is a product. The Durham rule was finally charged by the United States Attorney General's office with being capricious and burdensome—a charge that led eventually to its abandonment.

Details of these legal rules and the critical charges leveled against them should not obscure the central point. There is a moral reason for having available an insanity plea for offenders. Acts are defined as "criminal" by the system of criminal law. Yet those who commit criminal acts may be morally blameworthy or not, depending on their responsibility for the act. Those who are held responsible are deemed bad; their fate is then determined by the criminal justice system. Those held not responsible are the mad; they are considered in need of care, treatment, and rehabilitation. If the legal tests suffer from any inadequacies, they will probably fail to accomplish this humanitarian aim. To exculpate a criminal who should not be held responsible because he could not have acted otherwise represents a moral effort to make the way people are treated commensurate with the psychological determinants of their actions. The underlying assumption is that it is only just to punish those who are culpable for their actions. On this view, it is fair to apply the medical model and treat the criminally insane as patients. When such individuals pose a threat to society, they should be hospitalized, not jailed. There they can be given therapy or "rehabilitated," and released to the community when cured.

Defects in the Insanity Plea

A curious irony in practice has been that many people confined in institutions for the criminally insane have remained there for longer periods (sometimes up to a lifetime) than they would have spent in jail if given a lenient sentence or granted early parole. One general criticism that rests on these practical consequences indicts the insanity defense as being unduly harsh. The legal defense against criminal responsibility was intended to serve as a more humane alternative to indictment and incarceration, yet a discrepancy exists between the length of time criminal offenders remain incarcerated and the disproportionally longer periods of confinement experienced by mental patients. This is seen by some to be a moral failing of the insanity defense.

Another moral worry, this one of an opposing sort, is the fear that the insanity defense provides too lenient a way of treating criminal offenders. Psychopaths or neurotic offenders might escape responsibility for their criminal acts; yet they should, according to one view, be held responsible. This objection appeals both to considerations of justice and also to psychological assumptions about persons. It assumes that there is a significant difference between the responsibility that truly psychotic persons bear for their actions and that of a range of other people whose actions may nonetheless be psychologically determined. The ability of psychiatrists to make such discriminations in a systematic and uncontroversial manner has come under increasing attack. If there are to be alternative systems for determining the fate of allegedly different types of offenders against the criminal law, such alternatives must be based on clear criteria for separating them. Not only must these criteria rest on sound theoretical foundations in psychiatry and psychology; they must also be able to be applied consistently and knowledgeably in practice. All the rules governing the insanity defense employ wording that is not only vague but also differs substantially from the detailed technical terminology used for diagnostic purposes in clinical practice.

Taken together, all these objections have led in recent years to a call for the abolition of the insanity defense. Although the opposition to this legal option has risen sharply in the past twenty years or so, the difficulties had already been summarized over fifty years ago by Judge Benjamin Cardozo, who wrote:

> If insanity is not to be a defense, let us say so frankly and even brutally, but let us not mock ourselves with a definition that palters with reality. Such a method is neither good morals nor good science nor good law. [7]

Early in 1978, the New York State Department of Mental Hygiene recommended abolition of the insanity defense. The report charged psychiatrists with not being very good at determining who is legally insane. Oddly enough, the report held that prisons, rather than mental hospitals, are better equipped to care for the mentally ill who commit crimes. Still another reason cited in support of the recommendations was that those who are acquitted on grounds of insanity may be treated too leniently. The New York report called for a new rule—a "diminished capacity

---

[7]Benjamin N. Cardozo, *Law, Literature and Other Essays* (New York: Harcourt Brace, 1931), p. 3.

rule''—in which presence of an abnormal condition could lead to reduction in the severity of the crime. Under present law in this and other jurisdictions, those found not guilty by reason of insanity are detained in a mental hospital until it is determined that they can be released without danger to themselves or others.

These recent developments seem to reflect a loss of faith in psychiatric expertise regarding judgments of sanity or insanity. If the moral purposes behind distinguishing legally between the bad and the mad are to be served, those charged with making the distinction in practice must be capable of doing so consistently and accurately. If they cannot, or if the practice is subject to abuse, then a better system should be sought. To maintain the insanity defense in the face of sound scientific and practical objections would be to deceive the public into thinking psychiatrists possess some expertise that they lack. This is one kind of moral mistake in the practice of expert testimony.

A second kind of moral error lies in the potentially unfair results of the system: Like cases are not treated alike. If the system is too lenient, it may allow those who are truly responsible to succeed in being acquitted and to escape imprisonment. And, in contrast, it allows those who bear equal responsibility for their actions to be confined for significantly different periods of time, depending on whether they are imprisoned or committed to a mental institution. Arguments that charge the insanity defense with leading to unfairness have at least these two possible means of support, if not others. For these reasons, as well as shifting public opinion about personal responsibility, the humanitarian alternative to criminal guilt intended by the insanity defense seems now to be reversing itself. We turn next to a look at the proliferation of alternatives within institutions, both penal and mental.

Alternatives Within Institutions

One of the most effective and efficient ways to gain control over the behavior of those who are viewed as socially undesirable—for whatever reason—is to lock them up. At the very least, this achieves the result of keeping society's undesirables isolated from the mainstream of work and play. Over the centuries, treatment of inmates in institutions has ranged from what most people today would agree is brutal to what we hold repressive, consider tolerable, and even think humane. How inhabitants of institutions are treated is partly a function of the ethical beliefs and norms of behavior of a culture or of the particular group in charge of institutions. These beliefs and norms often change from one era or generation to the next.

There is yet another factor that determines what an inmate may be forced to undergo in a prison or mental hospital. The rather recent alternatives to traditional punishment are a product of advances in therapeutic technology. The development of psychiatry and clinical psychology over the past half century has given rise to the ''rehabilitative alternative''—an alternative to simply being institutionalized. To commit people to mental hospitals and to offer no treatment programs, and perhaps, therefore, no hope of release came to be known as ''warehousing.'' Before therapy was available as an alternative to punishment or mere confinement, there were few programs for treatment of inmates. The wedding of psychiatry and the law, along with the rise of technological means of behavior control, led to a series of curious developments, legally and morally.

One curiosity can be found in the apparent paradox that prisoners and mental patients alike, supported by their advocates, are claiming both the ''right to treatment" and the "right to refuse treatment." Objections to "warehousing," when therapeutic alternatives are available and viewed with hope, lead naturally to a call for treatment, expressed legally in terms of the "right to treatment." But there was a growing perception that many treatments administered under the guise of therapy—ECT, aversive conditioning through chemical control, and at the extreme, psychosurgery—were worse than no treatment at all. In just what respects they were perceived as "worse" is important for understanding the nature of the debate.

Another curious feature emerged from the availability of therapy as an alternative within institutions. That is the familiar difficulty arising out of the need to gain informed consent, this time with a new twist. As discussed earlier in connection with granting consent for psychosurgery, the problem with mental patients and the criminally insane is that "the damaged organ is the consenting organ." Court decisions mandating a "right to treatment" require that psychiatric patients not simply be warehoused. But if they are to be treated, it is usually necessary to go through the process of obtaining consent. It is not uncommon for psychiatric patients to be declared incompetent to grant consent. In these cases, it is normally a relative who signs the form authorizing treatment. When a procedure as invasive as psychosurgery or long-term drug therapy is proposed, there is serious concern that decisions made by anyone other than the subject infringe on the autonomy of the person whose moods and behavior are to be altered.

Alternatives within penal institutions include both standard treatments and research programs in which prisoners might participate. A number of research efforts have held out hope for benefiting the prisoner who chooses to be a subject. A notable example is the treatment of sex offenders by administering anti-androgens. These chemicals, which counteract male hormones, promise relief for the man who is caught in the grip of sexual drives beyond his understanding and control. If research programs yield fruitful results, both sex offenders and society at large stand to gain. Yet staunch opponents of the use of prisoners for biomedical and behavioral research hold that in spite of the likelihood of some benefits to prisoners themselves, it is morally wrong to use as "volunteers" those who, they claim, are incapable of giving fully voluntary consent. Calling any prisoners "volunteers" is a mere sham.

These moral issues have become a matter of public policy as society has directed attention toward the rights of prisoners and mental patients. Regulations have been embodied in guidelines at the federal level, as well as in state laws. Over the centuries, a dramatic shift has occurred in moral perceptions of what is permissible or obligatory in the treatment of institutionalized persons. In recent decades, proponents of the rehabilitative model have held that where effective therapy is believed to exist, failure to give treatment is inhumane. Viewed in this way, omitting treatment is similar to withholding penicillin or insulin where such drugs are known to be effective in combating bacterial infections or diabetes. Yet there is an equally forceful position that holds it inhumane to compel treatments, under the guise of therapy, when such methods are still in their experimental stages or are firmly rejected by patients. Even to make them available on a voluntary basis raises problems, since much doubt has been cast on the ability of any institutionalized persons to make fully voluntary choices.

It is understandable that a moral defense of the rights of inmates may support or reject rehabilitative programs in prisons. Some such programs have been judged inhumane with good reason. Courts have called them a form of "cruel and unusual punishment." One example of an invasive and frightening treatment is the use of the suffocating and paralyzing chemical, succinylcholine, in aversive conditioning programs (several programs are described more fully below). Some treatments have been openly experimental, such as the anti-androgen drug trials on prisoners who are sex offenders. Even if entered into voluntarily, it has been argued, no such programs ought be allowed.

The paradox of claims demanding the right to treatment and also the right to refuse treatment is obviously only an apparent paradox. Rights to treatment are claimed when the sought-after therapy is believed to be effective or truly rehabilitative. Rights to refuse treatment are claimed when methods are believed to be inhumane, too invasive, ineffective, or simply untested and therefore, of unproved worth. Increasingly, individuals are demanding the right to refuse treatment for no further reason than their wish not to be treated.

Behavior Modification in Prisons

Behavior modification programs in prisons provide an example that illustrates the chief ethical dilemmas and conflicts of value arising out of rehabilitative efforts. A set of experimental behavior modification programs in prisons was begun in the early 1970s. These were abandoned within a very few years, partially in response to charges that they violated the constitutional rights of prisoners. Some of these programs were voluntary, while others were involuntary. Apart from the enduring problem of whether or not prisoners are capable of granting voluntary consent, a key ethical question focused on the sorts of deprivations incarcerated persons underwent in these programs. Behavior modification programs known as "token economies" were set up so that prisoners had to earn tokens for acts of good behavior. The tokens earned could then be cashed in for goods or privileges. Objections arose when it became known that often, basic amenities of hygiene and comfort had to be earned by cashing in tokens. Were these token economies degrading and dehumanizing, as some people alleged? A brief description of some rehabilitative programs in prisons, along with objections raised against them, should supply some useful data.

> START (Special Treatment and Rehabilitative Training) was a Bureau of Prisons demonstration project for dealing with adult male offenders in long-term segregation begun in September 1972 at the Federal Medical Center in Springfield, Missouri. The designers of the project thought of it as a typical behavior modification program that rewarded good behavior rather than punished bad behavior. Located in a maximum security building, the program involved several different levels through which an inmate could progress, on the basis of a "good day" system in which he was rated in twelve different areas such as personal hygiene, conduct, politeness, and relations with the staff. Placement into the START program was from any other prison in the Federal system and was involuntary.[8]

Another involuntary program was CTP (Control Unit Treatment Program), set up by the Bureau of Prisons in the early 1970s. The purpose was to help inmates change

---

[8] "The Projects," p. 3. Unpublished research document prepared for a conference on Behavior Modification in Prisons, held at The Hastings Center in 1978. Tabitha M. Powledge did the research and wrote the reports as part of a project entitled "The Dynamics of Scientific Research: Three Case Studies of Scientific Research on Aggression," conducted by the Behavioral Studies Research Group. The project was supported by a grant from the EVIST Program of the National Science Foundation, grant OSS77-17072. Descriptions of the other treatment programs discussed in this section are also drawn from these research documents.

their attitude and behavior so that they could return to regular programs. In these programs, as in project START, transfer was involuntary. Prisoners seen as posing a threat to other inmates or staff were transferred from other forms of segregation. According to guidelines issued by the Bureau of Prisons, the CTP was to include counseling, a progression system through which the inmate could pass, and activities such as work, education, and recreation. The Bureau of Prisons claimed that the difference between START and the CTP programs was that the latter were intended chiefly for dangerous inmates who required close control. But when the Government Accounting Office conducted an evaluation in August 1975, they charged that the programs differed little, if at all, in their approach to modifying inmate behavior. CTP programs were in operation at Marion, a prison for young adults at El Reno, Oklahoma; Leavenworth, a young adult facility at Lompoc, California; and the prison at Milan, Michigan.

A voluntary program known as CMP (Contingency Management Program) was in operation for a brief period of time in the Virginia prison system. Administered by four psychology professors, this program used positive reinforcement techniques. It employed a token economy system in which inmates earned credits for "appropriate behavior," including personal hygiene, neatness, cooperation, and completing lessons. This program was refused further funding from the Law Enforcement Assistance Administration and was abandoned in the Fall of 1974.

When the existence and nature of these programs reached the attention of members of the United States Congress, a flurry of letters ensued. The Subcommittee on Courts, Civil Liberties and the Administration of Justice of the House Judiciary Committee inspected the prisons at Leavenworth and Springfield. In their report, the Subcommittee concluded that

> in many ways, the START program is no different than the segregation facilities located in other federal institutions.... The Subcommittee is of the opinion that methods of rehabilitation whose appropriateness are untested and questioned by reasonable people should not be forced upon individuals indiscriminately. Group therapy or chemico-psychological treatments or experimentation should not be required of those unwilling or unable to make an intelligent or free decision to submit to them. Additionally, there are very serious questions whether aspects of START violate the constitutional prohibition against cruel and unusual punishment.[9]

This judgment assesses a therapeutic effort by the standards of humane treatment that operate officially in the criminal justice system. The injunction against cruel and unusual punishment is a central moral feature of the penal law. It is not too surprising, then, to find an ethical precept operating in one institutional sphere being applied to a practice in a different area—in this case, rehabilitation. The line between therapy and social control becomes blurred once again when authorities apply the rules governing what is morally permissible in the realm of punishment to the therapeutic domain. One may even see behavior-modification programs in prisons as a way of legitimizing punishment in the name of science. Terms like "time-out rooms" are used to refer to "isolation rooms"; "no reinforcement" is used instead of "deprivation"; and "negative reinforcement" is employed in place of "punishment." Couching inhumane practices in a mantle of scientific respectability

---

[9] "The Federal Role in Prison Behavior Modification Programs," p. 10. Unpublished research document prepared by Tabitha M. Powledge (see footnote 6). This account presents a chronology of events from the mid-1960s through 1975, describing the Federal government's participation and the political opposition that developed.

appears to legitimate them, so that those in control are enabled to use techniques that would otherwise be prohibited.

The Right to Mental Autonomy

Why has the therapeutic alternative come to be seen as worse than outright punitive efforts? For one thing, cruel and unusual punishment has typically been construed as some form of bodily torture. But psychological torture may be even more devastating, since it typically aims at making inroads into the mind. The result may be a loss of the ability to think independently or form one's opinions freely and rationally. One way to express the moral wrong would be to refer to psychologically invasive techniques as intruding on a person's autonomy.

Protection of autonomy has been recognized legally in several court cases. The "right to mental autonomy" has been construed as a legally fundamental right ensuring "a person's power to generate thought, ideas, and mental activities—his freedom of mentation."[10] These considerations were evoked in a landmark psychosurgery case in Michigan (*Kaimowitz* v. *Michigan Department of Mental Health*), as well as in a case in California invoking a state prisoner who was administered succinycholine. The Kaimowitz court addressed the right to mental autonomy as follows:

> *A person's mental processes, the communication of ideas, and the generation of ideas come within the ambit of the First Amendment. To the extent that the First Amendment protects the dissemination of ideas and the expression of thoughts, it equally must protect the individual's right to generate ideas. . . .*[11]

In the California case, the plaintiff charged the defendants with "deliberate and malicious intentional infliction of mental and emotional distress." The court of appeals referred both to cruel and unusual punishment and to "impermissible tinkering with the mental processes."

Research on Prisoners

The introduction of therapy for inmates of institutions as an alternative to incarceration as punishment or warehousing has been unwelcome to many who have been subjected to these alternatives. Yet prisoners continue to demand the right to volunteer as research subjects, whether or not the research might stand to benefit them. One example is that of sex offenders, whose pleas for treatment the behavioral geneticist John Money takes seriously. Money writes:

> *Being arrested or in jail is a trauma that allows the sex offender to seek treatment. Ordinarily, sex offenders do not feel any more hurt or disabled because of their sex lives than do non-offenders. They know their behavior is socially stigmatized and punishable, but the threat of punishment is not traumatic enough to induce them to seek treatment. Thus, to fail to provide treatment at the time of arrest or imprisonment is, in most instances, to fail forever.*

[10]Paul R. Friedman, "Legal Regulation of Applied Behavior Analysis in Mental Institutions and Prisons," *Arizona Law Review* 17:1 (1975), pp. 58ff.

[11]*Ibid.*, p. 60.

The precedent for resolving the foregoing dilemma was established by a sex offender serving concurrent life sentences for rape and attempted rape. Recently he took his case to federal court and obtained an agreement from the prison authorities that they would make him available for treatment if he was accepted into the Johns Hopkins antiandrogen program. Then he received from the same judge a ruling that his consent to treatment was indeed informed consent: A physician and a psychologist informed him in the courtroom of the pros and cons of treatment. He has since been treated on a weekly basis in jail.[12]

This particular treatment program is an alternative offered to incarcerated criminals, which has met with strong objections at the hands of defenders of prisoners' rights. The debate over which side is in the right probably reduces quickly to one of those fundamental moral disagreements that admits of no rational resolution. One side claims that prisoners are not free to choose and so cannot grant truly voluntary consent to serve as research subjects. The other side argues minimally that prisoners have a degree of rational decision-making power sufficiently similar to most people who grant consent for research or therapy.

A different yet related view holds that further restriction of choices for those who possess barely any liberties at all can scarcely serve as an adequate moral defense against coercive practices. To protect prisoners against their own choices—however distorted—is a form of paternalism. Whether it is justified paternalism or not depends both on the moral premises one starts with and on the amount of freedom prisoners are believed to possess.

There is a crowning irony to this prisoner's dilemma. Either the types of behavioral research aimed at learning the causes of and remedies for aggressive and antisocial behavior must be abandoned altogether, thus removing all remaining hopes associated with rehabilitation for criminals; or else such experimental programs must be conducted on prisoners, if the requirements of "good science" are to be met. Any techniques for altering human behavior must undergo adequate testing before they can be honestly offered as accepted forms of therapy. Unlike a wide range of experiments—notably drug trials in biomedical research, where animals are used for experimentation before testing drugs on humans—in much behavioral research it makes no sense to conduct animal studies. Even when preliminary research on animals does make sense, as in experiments on aggression and testosterone levels, there comes a point where studies must be done on human subjects if research results are to be considered valid. The requirements of sound scientific methodology virtually dictate the use of a prison population for this purpose as best fulfilling the conditions of good research design. Those known to have committed crimes of violence are clearly the most appropriate subjects for research on criminal aggressive or violent behavior, as are sex offenders for research on criminal sexual aggression. Chronic offenders are more suitable as research subjects than first-time offenders, yet repeat offenders will have been incarcerated longer and as a result, are perhaps less capable of making free, voluntary choices to serve as research subjects.

There is no simple way out of this dilemma. On the one hand, it is morally questionable to use aversive conditioning routinely or to offer anti-androgens as therapy to prisoners or institutionalized psychiatric patients when such techniques

---

[12]John Money, "Issues and Attitudes in Research and Treatment of Various Forms of Human Sexual Behavior," in William H. Masters, Virginia E. Johnson, and Robert C. Kolodny, eds., *Ethical Issues in Sex Therapy and Research* (Boston: Little, Brown, 1977), p. 123.

have not undergone adequate testing. On the other hand, on whom but prisoners and mental patients can such research be conducted with optimal scientific validity? Good science virtually requires that those who have manifested undesirable social behavior regularly, frequently, and in the extreme, are the most appropriate subjects for experimental programs designed to control such behavior.

There is, finally, a political dimension to many of the ethical issues discussed in this chapter. Defenders of the rights of prisoners, mental patients, and other institutionalized persons often issue principled objections to all research programs proposed for these special populations. Or they may sometimes assert that the groups they seek to protect have a "right to treatment," and yet at other times demand their "right to refuse treatment." While these demands and assertions often rest on moral considerations, sometimes they arise out of political motives such as interest and power. When ideological factors become part of the debate, as they have in the deinstitutionalization movement of the last decade or so, it becomes even more difficult to identify the ethical issues clearly. The last section of this chapter takes up the question of alternatives to institutionalization—a subject of moral and political concern arising inevitably out of a clash between the hoped-for prospects and the unhappy results of efforts at deinstitutionalization.

Alternatives to Institutionalization

Nowhere is controversy fraught with more uncertainty about both facts and values than in the debates surrounding deinstitutionalization. Alternatives to institutionalization for special populations include a number of methods of behavior control already discussed as alternatives within institutions: physical manipulation of the brain, mood-altering drugs, implantation of electronic monitoring devices, physical or chemical castration of sex offenders. Despite the initial optimism that accompanied the deinstitutionalization movement, serious questions have emerged concerning the value tradeoffs. The reason it is hard to determine which of several alternatives is morally superior is twofold: (1) not enough is known about crucial facts—the long-term effectiveness of alternatives to institutionalization and the side-effects of medication and other invasive procedures; and (2) the chief values in conflict represent fundamentally different ethical principles or priorities.

Consider, for example, the value priorities involved in a principled debate over the more intrusive techniques used for altering the behavior of violent or aggressive persons. We have already reviewed the chief grounds for opposing invasive techniques that alter the brain physically by producing lesions in healthy tissue by surgically cutting out a portion of the brain, or by electrode stimulation. Yet many psychiatrists and neurosurgeons continue to argue for the use of these procedures on the grounds that such operations serve to benefit the person involved—"the patient," in the terminology of the medical model. If techniques such as psychosurgery, electrode implantation, and behavior-altering drugs do succeed in making violent or aggressive individuals conform to society's laws and moral rules, why should they not be considered preferable to the age-old method of putting people behind bars as a way of controlling their behavior?

It is no easy matter to decide which alternative is more coercive: keeping a criminal offender locked in a cell for twenty years or even for life; or performing a brain operation that has some likelihood of preventing future violent outbursts. Psychosurgery performed without the subject's prior consent seems to be the more coercive measure if emphasis is placed on both the reversibility of the method of behavior control and the effect of the procedure on the subject's autonomy. Psychiatrists seeking methods that lack these extreme features greeted with eager anticipation the emergence of antipsychotic medication, which held out promise for a humane alternative to indefinite incarceration of large numbers of mental patients. But the enthusiasm of psychiatrists for one major chemical alternative to institutionalization—the class of drugs known as phenothiazines—has waned considerably in the wake of increasing evidence that unpleasant and even irreversible side effects follow long-term use. An example is the frequent result of antipsychotic medication, known as "tardive dyskinesia," described more fully below.

There is no need to rehearse in detail the evils typical of total institutions. Excluding the brutalizing of inmates by guards or custodians, there remain the overly structured environment of prisons and mental hospitals, required conformity to schedules and regulations, severe limitations on freedom of movement, and the general "dehumanizing" effects of long-term residence. But as Gerald Klerman has observed:

> in the modern city, we also meet counterforces which suggest new limits to individuality; ironically, the price that individuals often pay for this potential freedom of choice is actual social isolation, personal loneliness, and the anomie that characterize so much of modern urban life, especially for the poor, the marginal, and the mentally ill. Thus the urban community may generate exactly the same psychological consequences that are likely to occur in a total institution. One of the unintended consequences of decarceration and deinstitutionalization may be new forms of anomie and isolation.[13]

The two principal positive reasons for maintaining these institutions also need to be borne in mind: their role in protecting society from allegedly dangerous persons; and the acknowledged paternalistic features of caring for those unable to care for themselves and protecting from self-destruction those likely to make successful suicide attempts.

There remains also the prospect of enhancing the autonomy of mental patients or the mentally retarded through behavior modification and other therapeutic programs in a controlled environment. Claims that cite alleged evils and presumed virtues of these and other rehabilitative efforts rest for their support on a mix of facts and values. Empirical evidence is available to demonstrate that institutions are, indeed, as dismal as they are often portrayed and also that the alternatives frequently fail to work as hoped for. Books and films abound—both fiction and documentary —depicting life in prisons and mental hospitals. Recent decades have witnessed newspaper exposés of horrendous conditions and brutalizing of inmates. So it is little wonder that a movement of sorts grew up among academics, political figures, advocacy groups, and the general public—a movement attacking total institutions in one respect or another, in whole or in part. The movement has sought release for members of various populations: the so-called mentally ill; those incarcerated for criminal offenses; the mentally retarded; the elderly.

But it is a confusing error to lump all these populations together when the aim is to seek alternatives to institutionalization on moral grounds. For one thing, the justifications offered for locking people up against their will differ strikingly, as we have already seen. But not only are there different justifications for housing deviant

<hr>

[13]Gerald Klerman, "Behavior Control and the Limits of Reform," *Hastings Center Report* 5 (August 1975), p. 45.

persons in total institutions; there are also different consequences that follow release into the community. One practical consequence has been the "dumping" of mental patients into localities—particularly as deinstitutionalization has been mandated by state laws—without providing money to care for them. There have also been disruptive effects on the communities themselves, with opposition often leading to the sad irony that former residents of total institutions gain their freedom at the expense of being feared or ostracized by members of the community where they take up residence. Following initial enthusiasm for the movement, deinstitutionalization has experienced a "backlash," especially in communities and neighborhoods opposed to halfway houses, smaller group residences, and day programs for released mental patients or the retarded.

In addition to state decrees requiring mental institutions to release patients who seem capable of functioning outside a hospital setting, there have been several Federal court decisions holding that mental patients are entitled to care in the "least restrictive" environment. The moral motives behind these judicial decisions are clear: "least restrictive" often means "least coercive," so a reduction in the amount of coercion an inmate must suffer is viewed as the morally preferable alternative. But when placed alongside another set of ethical standards, allowing people the benefit of the least restrictive environment may turn out to be a less preferable alternative on the whole. It is not only the visible spectre of shopping bag ladies wandering aimlessly about, sleeping in doorways and rummaging through garbage cans in search of food for survival, that haunts the seemingly humane alternative of deinstitutionalization. Nor is it the equally bleak picture of elderly persons lacking the will or the means to live in group homes or a family to support them, living in unheated vans, weak from malnutrition or illness, that chiefly compels a reordering of priorities. Instead, the emergence of some surprising, unintended consequences of the move to less restrictive alternatives, along with conceptual and moral uncertainty about the "lesser restrictiveness" of the most promising alternatives, demands a close examination of deinstitutionalization as the most humane alternative. There is little doubt that the purposes of deinstitutionalization, and the motives of those who support it, are humane: It is intended to provide greater freedom and autonomy to former inmates of total institutions. But only when deinstitutionalization policies were in place for a while, did it become evident that there were costs to be balanced against those gains in freedom and autonomy.

Deinstitutionalization of Willowbrook

The first example is the public health problem that arose following the Willowbrook consent decree. Willowbrook Developmental Center is a large facility for mentally retarded children and young adults, which became infamous as a result of a research program on viral hepatitis. Beginning around 1956 and continuing for at least fourteen years, experiments were carried out on retarded children whose parents granted consent for their deliberate injection of the virus by researchers studying the disease. Hepatitis was rampant among the residents of the institution, so the researchers defended the experiment by arguing that the children would almost certainly come down with the disease anyway, and that they would be better off in the carefully controlled circumstances provided by participation in a medical research program.

In an unrelated development, in 1975 a Federal court issued the Willowbrook consent decree, directing the state to care for the mentally retarded with certain staff ratios and in community surroundings. Quite apart from the events surrounding the hepatitis research conducted there, Willowbrook had gained notoriety as an example of an oversized, understaffed institution exhibiting squalor and inadequate methods of care and treatment of inmates. It is no wonder that it became a prime target for deinstitutionalization.

A concomitant of the deinstitutionalization movement has been the encouragement of "mainstreaming" retarded or learning-disabled children in public schools. While still recognizing the need for special training of and assistance to members of this population, proponents of mainstreaming have pointed to the enrichment and "normalization" that serve to benefit children who are not kept in segregated facilities. But following the gradual emptying of Willowbrook and the placement of former residents in public school classrooms, the discovery was made that a large number of these children were carriers of the hepatitis-B virus and could thus transmit the debilitating disease to healthy children.

By the late 1970s, this situation posed a significant dilemma for educators, public health officials, and those involved in carrying out the mandates of the Willowbrook consent decree. On the one hand, both the law and the humanitarian concerns behind the impetus to deinstitutionalize facilities such as Willowbrook required placement of former residents in a normal educational setting. On the other hand, the health hazard posed by the risk that carriers of a dread disease (for which no cure exists) might infect their classmates presents an ethical problem of a different sort. Two factors contribute to the problem. First is the unforeseen nature of this consequence of the Willowbrook deinstitutionalization. Second is the ethical dilemma posed by competing values in making a decision about where to place the retarded children who are carriers of hepatitis. The values in competition are on one side, utilitarian considerations involved in public health measures, and on the other side, the rights of individuals or special classes of persons (the mentally retarded, in this case). The decision to deinstitutionalize has Kantian moral roots, grounded in concern for the dignity and autonomy of persons—the inmates of institutions like Willowbrook. Decisions about hepatitis carriers appear to be public health matters, rather than ethical ones; but the utilitarian justification for instituting public health measures, which may infringe on the rights of individuals, appeals to the fundamental ethical principle mandating practices that offer the greatest benefit to the greatest number of people.

Side Effects of Antipsychotic Drugs

The second example of unforeseen consequences and moral uncertainty about alternatives is the emergence of a devastating side effect of antipsychotic drugs: the condition known as tardive dyskinesia. This neurological complication of long-term use of such drugs manifests itself in often grotesque, involuntary muscle movements of the face, mouth, and extremities. These movements may persist for years, even after the medication is discontinued. The symptoms usually do not develop until after a person has been taking the drug for months or even years, and by the time they appear it may be too late to reverse the condition. There is no known treatment that is satisfactory, and once it appears the condition is usually chronic.

This unforeseen side effect of antipsychotic medication is problematic for several reasons. First, it demonstrates that the effects of drugs as well as procedures such as psychosurgery can be irreversible and undesirable. This discovery offers cause to doubt the validity of making sharp distinctions between drugs and more invasive methods of behavior control. Secondly, the development of thorazine and similar drugs has been hailed as providing a less restrictive alternative for seriously ill patients than indefinite confinement in a total institution. There is reason to question that earlier optimism now that the values in the risk-benefit equation are more clearly defined. What value should be placed on a method of controlling behavior that leads to remission of psychotic symptoms but substitutes uncontrollable neurological ones?

Finally, the emergence of tardive dyskinesia serves as a reminder that few medical therapeutic interventions are free of untoward consequences. It is reasonable to expect that the development of other new drugs will be accompanied by side effects of their own, thereby diminishing the prospects that a clear value priority will emerge between institutionalization and its alternatives.

There is, then, ample reason to question the supposition that total institutions comprise the "most restrictive" alternative among the available choices for controlling the behavior of society's deviant or helpless members. Whether it is the physical or chemical castration of sex offenders proposed as an alternative to imprisonment; sterilization of mentally retarded young women as an alternative to keeping them isolated at home or in an institution; or simply releasing mentally ill or retarded or elderly persons into the community, so that they must use their newfound freedom to fend for themselves or perish, the difficulty of arriving at a clear and uncontroversial judgment is apparent. While physical confinement in a total institution is a dramatic mode of limiting freedom, invading privacy, and subverting autonomy, it is surely not the only or, perhaps, even the morally worst method.

Potential for Abuse

A final issue to consider is the potential for abuse. In 1974, the *Los Angeles Times* reported an interest on the part of public officials in using new technological approaches for the purpose of screening, predicting, keeping under surveillance, and actually controlling the behavior of violence-prone individuals and groups. The article cited a proposal to attach miniature tracking devices called "transponders" to arrestees and criminals as a condition of parole. A member of the National Security Agency suggested that these devices could be used for "monitoring aliens and political subgroups" as well. Fears about the technological potential for controlling behavior go hand in hand with a growing mistrust of those in whose hands the research and development of such controls will inevitably fall. This raises the broader social issue of behavior control in a free society. What should the role of psychiatrists be in contributing to research efforts whose outcomes may be instruments of broad social control or possible tools for oppression of political dissidents, minority agitators, or social reformers? The preceding chapter explored these issues as they relate to therapy versus social control in the Soviet Union, a country fundamentally lacking many of the freedoms Westerners enjoy. The next chapter takes a look at a number of episodes that raise similar ethical questions about the activities of some psychiatrists and psychologists in our own society.

FURTHER READINGS

FINGARETTE, HERBERT, *The Meaning of Criminal Insanity*. Berkeley: University of California Press, 1972.

GOLDSTEIN, ABRAHAM S., *The Insanity Defense*. New Haven: Yale University Press, 1967.

MURPHIE, JEFFRIE G., ed., *Punishment and Rehabilitation*. Belmont, California: Wadsworth Publishing Company, 1973.

NATIONAL COMMISSION FOR THE PROTECTION OF HUMAN SUBJECTS, *Research Involving Prisoners: Report and Recommendations* and *Appendix*. Washington, D.C.: U.S. Department of Health, Education, and Welfare, 1976.

_____, *Research Involving Those Institutionalized as Mentally Infirm: Report and Recommendations* and *Appendix*. Washington, D.C.: U.S. Department of Health, Education, and Welfare, 1976.

ROTHMAN, DAVID, *The Discovery of the Asylum: Social Order and Disorder in the New Republic*. Boston: Little, Brown and Co., 1971.

CHAPTER 6

Behavior Control in a Free Society: Treatment and Research

'You've sinned, I suppose, but your punishment has been out of all proportion. They have turned you into something other than a human being. You have no power of choice any longer. You are committed to socially acceptable acts, a little machine capable only of good. . . . A man who cannot choose ceases to be a man. . . . To turn a decent young man into a piece of clockwork should not, surely, be seen as any triumph for any government, save one that boasts of its repressiveness.'

ANTHONY BURGESS
A Clockwork Orange

They worked on ways to achieve the "controlled production" of headaches and earaches; twitches, jerks and staggers. They wanted to reduce a man to a bewildered, self-doubting mass to "subvert his principles," a C.I.A. document said. They wanted to direct him in ways that "may vary from rationalizing a disloyal act to the construction of a new person."

The New York Times, Aug. 2, 1977

The Issues

Following decades of hope and promise concerning scientific progress, the past ten years or so have witnessed a decline in optimism and a mounting mistrust on the part of the public of scientific experts. This is no less true in the field of behavior control than in areas such as nuclear energy development, the conquest of outer space, or the discovery of low-risk, high-benefit drugs and medical procedures. One consequence of this increased skepticism about the work of biomedical and behavioral scientists has been a greater demand for public participation in decision making at various levels. Another result has been a proliferation of commissions and boards to study and report on ethical practices. The National Research Act of 1974 brought into existence the National Commission for the Protection of Human Subjects of Biomedical and Behavioral Research. Its charge was to develop ethical guidelines for the conduct of research involving human subjects and to make recommendations for the application of such guidelines. Among the special populations on which the National Commission reported were prisoners and the institutionalized mentally infirm. That Commission disbanded upon fulfillment of its charge in 1978, but was replaced immediately by a newly formed body, the President's Commission for the Study of Ethical Problems in Medicine and Biomedical and Behavioral Research. Also brought into existence in the late 1970s was a body within the Department of Health and Human Services—the Ethics Advisory Board, which conducted hearings on developments in the biomedical arena and served in an advisory capacity to the Secretary of DHHS.

This chapter raises a number of questions about decision making in the public policy sector of behavior control. The questions are similar, whether the decisions affect a local community, a special population, or the populace as a whole. The discussion here is set against a backdrop of the political system in the United States—one characterized by the ideals of freedom and democracy and committed to the resolution of pressing social issues through the political process. The philosophical work of settling knotty moral issues is hard enough; it is yet another overwhelming task to succeed in getting the best moral solution implemented in practice.

How much public participation should a democratic society promote in decisions that raise issues of behavior control? The answer to this question is neither clear nor simple. But the question invites serious thought both about the justifiable limits of behavior control interventions and about the role of the public in determining policy. Where members of the psychiatric profession act as agents of social control, the role of the public inevitably becomes an issue. Two such cases are explored later in this chapter. The first case surrounds a proposed center for the purpose of doing research on the causes and control of violence. The center was to be connected with the Neuropsychiatric Institute at UCLA, but failed to open because of public outcry and protests by civil liberties spokesmen. The second case is that of recently disclosed CIA investigations into techniques of mind control and brainwashing, in which psychiatrists and psychologists cooperated. Both cases raise fundamental questions about behavior control in a free society: What is the proper social role of psychiatrists and other mental health specialists regarding such activities? Do the requirements of general utility override respect for the dignity and autonomy of individual patients or research subjects? Does psychiatric expertise automatically carry with it authority to engage in behavior control efforts in the broader social sphere?

The notion of expertise embodies one crucial concern both in scientific or technical domains and in the moral sphere. In a democratic society, the general presumption must be in favor of reaching decisions by democratic political processes. Nevertheless, notable circumstances occur where the presumption is likely to lie against decisions being made by the public, and in favor of decision making by experts. Aside from obvious cases such as day-to-day matters requiring rapid, continuous choices at various government levels—cases that could not reasonably employ modes of public participation—a large number of decisions remain in which optimal solutions require people with expert knowledge. In some situations this may simply demand thorough acquaintance with the facts. But in addition to knowing factual details about the cases at hand, there is a further sort of expertise that may be required—the kind that comes from special training, clinical experience, or advanced education. Here is where the notion of expertise impinges on the question of whether the approach to behavior control issues in society should follow democratic patterns.

Who are the experts in the area of behavior control? The obvious answer is those with special training, clinical experience, or advanced education, namely, psychiatrists and psychologists. Although this point has been contested both by laypersons and some of these alleged experts themselves, let us begin by granting it. Assume there is a body of knowledge and experience that mental health professionals have that those not trained or educated in these fields lack. But whatever this area of expertise may be, it surely does not cover all instances of decision making in the social domain of behavior control. Some decisions may be matters for scientific or technical expertise, since they require predicting the probable results and possible side effects of a technique such as psychosurgery or electrode implantation. Others may be partly or even largely matters of what is socially desirable or morally right, such as the conditions under which psychosurgery may ethically be performed, or whether electronic surveillance devices should be implanted in the brains of parolees. Are those whose expertise lies in the field of psychology or psychiatry especially equipped to make these value-laden decisions, as well? Does scientific or technical expertise confer authority on someone to make socially significant decisions having a major moral component? It seems reasonable to think not, since technical expertise lies in knowledge of relevant facts and scientific theories, while something else is at stake when behavior control decisions encompass social and ethical values.

Now an age-old question rises to the fore: Is there such a thing as *moral* expertise? Once again, two opposing sides are locked in debate. In order for there to be moral experts, moral knowledge has to be possible. There must be moral truths and ways of coming to know them. Whether or not the notion of moral knowledge is defensible has long been a subject of debate among philosophers—debate too large and complex to explore here. Opponents of the view that there are objective moral truths and sound methods for coming to know them would reject the idea that there could be any sort of moral expertise. If there is no body of moral knowledge, then what could possibly be the object of moral expertise?

Plato, taking the other side, was one of the first—but surely not the last—to hold that moral knowledge is no different from genuine knowledge of any other kind, including scientific knowledge. Those with the capacity and training to apprehend truths—moral or otherwise—will eventually come to know the good. For

Plato, knowledge of all other values depends first and foremost on knowledge of the good. But Plato never really explains just what constitutes the good, and this crucial point remains the center of debate. The problem is especially acute in a pluralistic society, where tolerance for a variety of preferred values is encouraged and usually practiced.

The proper role of psychiatry in decisions having an inevitable value component must be faced squarely. Whether the decisions encompass broad social policies or arise as part of the individual therapist-patient relationship, they emerge as ethical issues in the control of human behavior in a free society. Whoever may actually decide such issues and whatever the content of the decisions they reach, it remains unclear whether anything like moral expertise is involved. Suppose there is no such thing as a moral expert. Should social and political decisions concerning behavior control be left in the hands of those who are experts in behavior control? The harder it is to provide a convincing account of what a moral expert is, the more it would seem that decision making should follow democratic processes in a society committed to that political ideology. Granted, many policy decisions require considerable expertise of the technical kind, so laypersons will not understand all the necessary facts and theories required for knowledgeable policy making. But if there is strong interest in preserving public participation in decisions having a moral and social impact, then a practical way of handling this problem will be sought and adopted here, as in other areas where complex or highly technical matters are presented to the public for their understanding and debate.

In institutional psychiatry, conflicting loyalties may pose moral dilemmas for a psychiatrist employed by the military or a university or a state hospital. Is it the psychiatrist's duty, as a physician, always and only to serve the interests of his patient? Or does being in the employ of an institution—medical or otherwise—set up a new set of obligations a psychiatrist must honor? From such conflicting loyalties arise a host of moral dilemmas that have been dubbed "double agent" problems. The next section will explore at greater length the issue of duty conflicts as they arise in the clinical practices of psychiatry and psychology. While such moral dilemmas are found in medical practice wherever a doctor or therapist is employed by an organization or institution—diagnosing and treating patients as part of his job—the ethical dimensions take on special meaning in the area of behavior control.

The Psychiatrist as "Double Agent"

A spy who serves two warring states is the classic example of the double agent. He has obligations to two different factions—factions whose interests are starkly opposed. Less portentous than an actor in a drama of international intrigue but nonetheless a significant figure in the lives of those he affects, is the psychiatrist employed by an institution. The institution may be a prison, a university, or the military. It may be a mental hospital—public or private. In a broader sense of "institution," psychiatrists may choose or be called on to serve the largest possible organization in society possessing the power to affect people's liberty: the government itself.

Whatever the size or character of the institution, psychiatrists employed in such settings are beset with an ongoing dilemma: Whom do they serve? The institution that employs them? Or the individual who is diagnosed and treated—the patient, in the ordinary medical sense? What are the moral claims on the psychiatrist in such a situation? Whose interests should take precedence when they come into conflict? If the international spy does not confront an insoluble dilemma of double agency, it is because he usually "really" works for one government or the other when he acts as double agent. So might the psychiatrist in fact have clear priorities when interests clash. But this does not solve the moral issue: To whom *ought* psychiatrists be loyal when they face conflicting duties? This set of ethical issues can be classed under the heading "moral problems for the psychiatrist as double agent."

Most double-agency situations are best viewed from the moral point of view as cases of conflict of loyalty or clashes of duty, both of which cannot be performed simultaneously. One psychiatrist describes the situation as follows:

> *The psychiatrist or any other professional in the double-agent situation always has a dilemma when he is not in concordance with the values of the agency. The typical example conjured up is the psychiatrist in the military who feels a tension with the stated grounds of the military at a particular historical moment, like the Vietnam war.*
>
> *Consider the alternative situation where the psychiatrist is ideologically in agreement with the military, as were many psychiatrists in World War II. For those people there was no doubt that the psychiatrist had a moral obligation to the society; for them that moral obligation may have had a higher moral value than the obligation to the distressed single individual. For the military psychiatrist it was not a question of being an agent of an immoral or nonmoral situation, it was a dilemma between two moral commitments: loyalty to a set of values threatened in a wartime situation and loyalty to the value of treating individuals who may or may not be in distress. The double-agent problem is qualitatively different, depending upon whether the psychiatrist is committed to a moral situation.[1]*

It is not clear to begin with whether there is one right answer to the question: Whom ought military psychiatrists primarily serve—their patients or the military? Some espouse the radical view that military establishments are inherently unjust institutions. Their answer to the question would probably express the underlying moral assumption that when actions defy military authority or sabotage the system, they are justifiable. Others would argue just as forcefully that some wars, such as World War II, not only are justly fought but that they must be fought for reasons of group survival as well as for preservation of a way of life. Their answer to the double-agent question would most likely depend on the particular war and other related circumstances. Still others will assert that the demands of the society always take precedence over those of the individual, so that the psychiatrist's duty is first to the group, then to the patient, whether the war is a just one or not. This utilitarian position need not be limited to the practice of psychiatry in wartime, but has been used to justify activities such as psychological research in support of CIA efforts in time of peace, as well.

Military Psychiatry: A Case Study

To fix ideas, let us focus on a case study of military psychiatry in peacetime. In the case to follow, the psychiatrist was not being asked as part of his job to diagnose and treat conditions (whether they are called illnesses or not) whose

---

[1]Gerald L. Klerman, "In the Service of the State: The Psychiatrist as Double Agent," *Hastings Center Report* 8 (April 1978), p. 4.

presence is relevant to the very purpose of the military, the conduct of war. Being a homosexual does not hinder a soldier's efforts to do what he is expected to do in the military, and that posed a moral problem in the following case.

A young psychiatrist doing required military service was stationed in a remote Pacific location for one year. The United States military base was fairly far from cities or recreational areas and there was no war or other relevant military activity in progress. With regularity, authorities on the base sent military personnel for a psychiatric evaluation of their sexual orientation, seeking to discover whether they were homosexuals. The psychiatrist initially could not decide how to respond and remained in a quandary, early in his stay, about how to deal with these requests. Eventually he developed a strategy for dealing with what he was being asked to do. He agreed to perform psychiatric evaluations when ordered (since that was, in fact, his job), but refused to comment on the individual's sexual status unless, in his professional judgment, there was psychiatric illness present *and* the illness was functionally related to homosexuality. In addition, he always told the men sent to him exactly what his evaluation to the authorities would be. This psychiatrist's frank admission—after reflecting for some time—was that the task of evaluating soldiers as homosexuals simply was not part of his job as a psychiatrist.[2]

It was hard for this young psychiatrist to think through the problem in a clear way when these requests first began, since nothing in his medical education or psychiatric training had prepared him for the role he was forced to adapt to. Once he formed the value judgment that what the military authorities were asking him to do was outside the bounds of proper professional practice, he then had to use his ingenuity to develop an appropriate response. The psychiatrist never was fully informed about the reasons why all these requests for homosexual evaluations were forthcoming, yet he was aware that those requesting the sexual status evaluations took a dim view of homosexuals, so his own compliance might result in specific harms to some soldiers. It is worth noting that this psychiatrist thought his own theoretical position on homosexuality—whether it is a psychiatric disease or not—was quite irrelevant to the moral dilemma into which he was thrust. Other psychiatrists would have come to a different decision about what to do; some probably would not have perceived any ethical conflict at all in the situation.

The psychiatrist in this situation later realized that much of his initial confusion stemmed from trying to distinguish what he knew as an expert from what the military was willing to accept he knew.

> They often wanted me, as an authority, to say things beyond my expertise. For example, I had no professional way to identify a homosexual, yet the Marine Corps would have gladly added my opinion to their evidence in such a case. The only way that I, as a psychiatrist, could be helpful would be to use my authority and role as a professional to obtain information. This would involve dishonesty towards the patient and the military. To the patient I would be obtaining information falsely under the guise of being an interested expert, and to the military I would be pawning off personal judgment under the guise of expert opinion. I chose instead to delineate those areas I could not know and address myself to what I could know: the presence or absence of psychopathology.[3]

[2]This story was reported in personal conversation with the author by Howard Fenn, M.D., the psychiatrist who experienced the dilemma.

[3]Howard Fenn, correspondence with the author.

This case study portrays a scene in military psychiatry where the fear of losing life or limb, often operating in wartime, is absent and thus does not distort the dilemma of double agency.

School Psychiatry: A Case Study

It is useful to cite a somewhat different example, a case involving school psychiatry, to illustrate another ethical aspect of double-agent problems.

> A young first year medical student was having a severe emotional crisis. Obviously on the verge of a complete breakdown, he went to a private psychiatrist. He was agitated, anxious, didn't know if he could handle his studies. He had a brilliant college record, and clearly outstanding intellectual capacity.
>
> He was in acute distress and seemingly in the process of disintegration. The psychiatrist, trying very hard to avoid hospitalization, started intensive psychotherapy. The student was already at a point where it looked like he was going to have a schizophrenic break: reality testing was impaired, ideas of reference were occurring, and a hypomanic mood with grandiose ideation was forming. To relieve the pressures on him the psychiatrist wrote a letter for him saying that he was treating the student for "emotional problems" and recommended a medical leave of absence.
>
> The next fall the student attempted to return to medical school but was refused readmission, even though the psychiatrist had written a letter, as the physician in charge of the treatment, that he was medically able to continue his studies. They gave no reason for not reinstating him except that he was not considered suitable. He then began to apply to other medical schools at his psychiatrist's suggestion and was refused in every case. Before seeing the private psychiatrist the student had consulted the school psychiatrist who made a diagnosis of latent schizophrenia.
>
> When other medical schools wrote to his former school, the reason for discharge was medical leave with latent schizophrenia. It is known that about half of those with schizophrenia in remission will have another break. In the case of this student there was a real risk to future patients. He was planning to become a surgeon. The combination of a grandiose self-appraisal with the power of a surgeon could cause serious harm.
>
> The private psychiatrist recognized that there may be psychiatric conditions which would interfere with a career in medicine and therefore might be grounds for exclusion from medical school. The problem, as he saw it, was whether the school psychiatrist was seeing the student in his role as psychiatrist or in his role as part of the school administration, and whether these two roles could be separated.[4]

Conflicting Roles of Institutional Psychiatrists

Double-agency problems such as this are almost inevitable features of institutional psychiatry. A straightforward conflict occurs between two different social roles—roles that pose no moral dilemmas when they exist alone. An employee of an institution normally has—or ought to have—some loyalty to the employer. Whether this loyalty takes the form of refusing to impart industrial product information to competitors or defending the institution in public places, there is a reasonable expectation that working for an organization carries some commitment to what it stands for and a willingness to defend it. Often, there are specific obligations that

---

[4] "The Psychiatrist as Double Agent," *Hastings Center Report* 4 (February 1974), p. 12.

are based on contract. At other times, the duties of an employee derive from a structural hierarchy of authority within an organization. There are, of course, notable and justifiable exceptions. When people face virtual enslavement at the hands of their employers, and there are no alternative opportunities for work, forms of disloyalty designed to better their condition could be defended by sound moral arguments. A general presumption of loyalty is not an absolute one. Like most guides to moral action, general rules have notable exceptions.

Psychiatrists must come to grips with conflicting loyalties, however. Especially since they are educated as physicians and socialized into the medical profession, as well as trained in the specialty of psychiatry, there is an overwhelming moral force behind the dictates of keeping patients' confidentiality and respecting their privacy. Problems of double agency are not confined to the psychiatric branch of medicine, however. Doctors who work for institutions such as schools or prisons are likely to face many instances of conflicting loyalties. As physicians are employed more and more by industry and by insurance companies, moral dilemmas of this sort will arise with ever greater frequency. Yet the problem seems more profound in psychiatry, in part because successful therapy often depends on maintaining a relationship of trust between therapist and patient. Another reason is that the psychiatrist in an institution is frequently looked to as an agent of social control, unlike the ordinary doctor in most settings. Psychiatrists in mental hospitals have to confront patient management problems that constantly plague the regular attending staff. Equipped with powerful tools in the form of antipsychotic medication and electroconvulsive therapy, psychiatrists have the capacity to alter radically their patients' behavior as well as their moods. Add to that their medical authority in the hospital setting, and it is easy to see how psychiatrists become—wittingly or unwittingly—agents of social control in institutions. The situation is even more pronounced in prisons, perhaps because there is little or no presumption of sickness (or else the inmate would be in a medical rather than a penal institution).

It is not surprising that psychiatrists achieve legitimate authority in mental hospitals. The power they wield might be considered justifiably exercised. They are, after all, the experts in emotional and behavioral disorders. If there is a valid notion of psychiatric expertise, then psychiatrists—at least good ones—must be the ones to possess it. If, as some have argued, mental illness is a myth and, consequently, there is no subject matter about which to be an expert, then any argument defending psychiatrists' place of authority in mental institutions—based on their alleged expertise—may lose its soundness. But continuing to accept the premises with which we began, let us assume there is some body of knowledge concerning the cause and cure of human emotional and behavioral disorders. While acknowledging this does not eliminate moral dilemmas arising out of conflict of loyalty to institutional employer and to the patient, there is nonetheless more reason to grant psychiatrists a role of authority and expertise in this type of institution than in settings unrelated to the diagnosis and treatment of psychopathology.

In prisons, the role of psychiatrists may remain systematically ambiguous. Prisoners do not have the normal characteristics of patients. In most cases, prisoners do not think they are mentally ill, nor are they diagnosed as such. One psychiatric viewpoint nonetheless holds that anyone capable of committing the violent, horrible deeds performed by many criminal offenders could not possibly be normal, sane, or healthy. This position is not convincing as it stands, however, especially in the absence of a personality theory or a theory of psychopathology on which to base judgments about violent or antisocial behavior. This view aside, there may still be a legitimate role for psychiatrists in prisons when treatment programs exist. As described in the previous chapter, behavior modification and other attempts at psychological rehabilitation have been introduced in prisons. To the extent that these remain and show some success as therapy, the situation bears some similarity to the doctor-patient relationship in mental hospitals. Yet the psychiatrist is likely to serve as an agent of social control anyway, because of the primary function of penal institutions.

Even though the role of prison psychiatrists is ambiguous in these ways, moral presumptions still govern their behavior. Psychiatrists acting as agents of social control in prison settings are more likely using their authority than using their expertise. There is relatively little agreement on the causes of violence. Strong arguments have been advanced in support of the view that violent behavior has primarily social and environmental causes rather than being a pathological condition within a person that warrants psychiatric management. Whatever the correct explanation for the actions of violent criminal offenders, behavior control in prisons confronts the psychiatrist with problems of conflicting duties: to the prisoners who end up becoming patients, and to the employing institution.

Approaches to Resolving Problems of Double Agency

What solutions are promising for moral problems of double agency in behavior control? In addition to specific strategies like the one the young psychiatrist on the military base worked out for himself, three different approaches cover the basic options in this range of cases.

The first approach—not always possible to adopt—is for a psychiatrist or psychologist to avoid such conflicts by refusing to work in a situation that gives rise to them. The hardest one to avoid is obviously the military, as long as virtually all physicans are required to serve. Mandatory military service aside, practicing psychiatrists voluntarily enter most other institutional settings. With enough foreknowledge and sufficient concern, psychiatrists could deliberately shun this type of employment as a matter of policy. But would this yield the happiest solution? There would almost surely be a genuine loss of quality in therapeutic and counseling services if psychiatrists and psychologists who are most sensitive to ethical issues and conflicts of duty were to make themselves unavailable for such employment. It is often remarked that the quality of institutional psychiatry is considerably lower than the level found among private practitioners in urban settings and psychiatrists in teaching hospitals. If those already sensitive to moral concerns were to shrink from employment in educational and penal institutions, the moral dilemmas would not go away. They would remain, at worst, unrecognized; at the least, unheeded.

A radically different approach might be taken by psychiatrists who choose to work for an organization or institution, as well as by all who must serve time in the military. In this view, institutional psychiatrists should not really consider the people they treat as patients, in the usual sense implied by the doctor-patient relationship. Instead, psychiatrists in the employ of institutions should think of their seeming patients as impaired creatures sent by a different official for some sort of treatment—much as you might take a broken machine to the repair shop. This may sound crass, but it is an attitude not unheard of in prisons, according to some observers. Like the first approach, this method deals with the double-agent problem by trying to make it go away. To urge that the psychiatrist ought always serve the organization he is employed by, rather than show primary loyalty to the individual sent to him as a patient, is to take an ideological stance with few sound reasons behind it.

The third approach amounts to a form of compromise. A solution suggested by some psychiatrists who came together to grapple with these very issues was for the therapist to issue something akin to a "Miranda warning" in potential double-agent settings. Just as a policeman apprehending a suspect is required to inform the captive of his legal rights—most importantly, warning that anything he says may be held against him—so might a psychiatrist act in institutional settings. Recognizing that there is always a strong presumption favoring a doctor's primary loyalty to his patient, these psychiatrists realistically acknowledged that there are times when the moral presumption may legitimately lie elsewhere. The use of a "psychiatric Miranda warning" succeeds in confronting the potentially conflicting roles some psychiatrists may be forced to embrace as well as or better than any other policy for dealing with clashes of duty. Individual resolutions of particular double-agent dilemmas will differ in their fine points. But telling a patient that what he says may be held against him has at least the virtue of honesty. A large part of what is wrong with the questionable moral practice of breaking patients' confidentiality is ignoring or dashing their legitimate and justified expectations. If expectations become changed, by the use of something like a psychiatric Miranda warning, then the moral presumptions regarding confidentiality and privacy shift slightly from what they would be in the usual therapist-patient relationship. According to some practitioners, however, adopting this procedure might have the unwanted effect of undermining therapeutic prospects. In addition, some psychiatric patients could hardly be expected to assess such "Miranda warnings" correctly. Those who are less than fully competent stand in need of greater protection than the typical adult who is presumed rational and autonomous.

This device could not hope to resolve all duty conflicts or competing loyalties in behavior control any more than other rather simple solutions proposed for knotty moral problems. It may, however, force psychologists and psychiatrists who are employees of an institution to face squarely the matter of their priorities. It is one thing to adhere somewhat vaguely to the dictates of patient privacy and confidentiality while serving as an employee of an organization with its own agenda. It is quite another thing to have to decide, in diagnosing and treating patients, just what warnings or information should be imparted to whom and why. The prison psychiatrist may hope to serve the interests of criminal justice and also try to rehabilitate hardened criminals. The school psychiatrist may take the students' wishes and desires to heart, while continuing to maintain the goals and purposes of the educational institution. It is often hard, in practice—if not impossible, in principle—to do both simultaneously.

Behavior-Control Research

Few would contest the importance of gaining increased knowledge about the causes and control of violent or antisocial behavior. Only a few oppose psychiatric research efforts of any sort; but a large number of people express grave doubts about the design and implementation of neuropsychiatric studies whose aim is to understand and predict violent behavior. Some of these doubts arise out of a consideration mentioned earlier: a prevalent view that the reasons behind acts of violence lie in social circumstances rather than within the individual. Other objections are tied more closely to the nature of the research itself, claiming not that there is no knowledge to be gained by such investigations but that knowledge gained by these means is likely to be at the expense of the individuals' safety, privacy, or autonomy. Further fears stem from possible abuses that may occur during research efforts or in attempts to apply their results.

Violent and antisocial behavior remains a matter of deep concern to the public and its elected representatives. A recent *New York Times* article bore the headline "House Panel on Violent Crime Finds Experts Are Short on Solutions." The panel in question was a House of Representatives subcommittee holding hearings in Manhattan on the subject of violence. The subcommittee's responsibility was to oversee investigations on the effectiveness of current federal research efforts into violent behavior and sexual assault.

The *Times* article stressed how little is still known about the fundamental causes of violent behavior, even after a decade of federally sponsored research. A University of Pennsylvania sociologist testified before the subcommittee that "the weight of empirical evidence indicates that no current preventative [sic], deterrent, or rehabilitative intervention scheme has the desired effect of reducing crime."[5] Holding one popular viewpoint, several criminologists urged stiffer sentences for those considered "hard-core criminals" and fixed sentences with no possibility of time off for good behavior for others. On the opposing side, one witness argued that such deterrence strategies erred in assuming that potential offenders will weigh the costs and thus act "rationally." The report concluded by noting that criminological research is increasing, spurred by federal grants. Yet the result of research, according to the House subcommittee chairman, has been largely to demonstrate "how far we still are from solving the crime problem."

A natural response to a report of this kind would be to conclude that what is needed is even more research on the causes and effective prevention of violence. Skeptics might come to the opposite conclusion, however, based on the singular lack of success to date of virtually all efforts to understand and control violent behavior. Among the more bizarre social and political developments in recent years have been a number of controversies that erupted over research and treatment programs in the area of violence. Some of these were controversial programs involving prisoners, of the sort described in the preceding chapter—programs using techniques of aversive conditioning or token economies, which were dubbed "cruel and unusual punishment." Others focused on research efforts outside the prison setting, attempting to gain a better understanding of "crime in the streets."

When conflicts occur over research on human violence, they often involve a mix of ethical, social, and political elements. Particularly when research programs become known to the public, a variety of concerns are voiced by special interest groups as well as by advocates of civil liberties generally. A striking example of the interplay of these factors is the series of episodes surrounding the attempt to establish a Center for the Study and Reduction of Violence at the Neuropsychiatric Institute of the University of California at Los Angeles.

Some of the general themes addressed in earlier chapters resound clearly in the events between 1972 and 1974 in California. These themes also run through the broader issues surrounding research on violence and antisocial behavior, under

---

[5]Marvin E. Wolfgang, quoted in *The New York Times*, Jan. 15, 1978, p. 34.

whatever auspices such research is conducted. Two ideas discussed earlier reemerge in the present context: the issue of therapy versus social control, and the medical or disease model as a way of conceptualizing and treating violent behavior.

Justifying Research on Violence

To ask about the purpose for which research on violence is conducted is to raise a question about therapy versus social control. For whose benefit is such research intended? Is it for the actual or potential offender, who is considered sick, evil, or deficient in some way? Or is it for the good of the public at large to protect the innocent from potentially dangerous individuals? The likely answer to this set of questions is "both." A preliminary draft describing the proposed UCLA Center includes the remark: "No one claims that all violent persons have abnormally functioning brains. However, it is essential to discover those individuals who are so afflicted in order that corrective and preventive measures can be undertaken for their own protection and for the safety of society." An additional concern focuses more specifically on the long-range goals of research on violence. Is the eventual aim to change the behavior of actual offenders? Or to divert those judged as potentially violent from aggressive, antisocial behavior, and, if so, by what means?

Whether or not it is appropriate to think of these issues in terms of the medical model requires a look at some assumptions about the nature of violence underlying research of this type. To undertake neurophysiological and biochemical investigations of people who have committed violent acts clearly presupposes the validity of a biological explanation of behavior in these contexts. Such research seeks the causes of violent behavior within the individual, not only at a psychological level of functioning but from a "deeper" source: a person's neurological and endocrinological or hormonal functions. There is little doubt that investigating neurobiological causes of behavior falls squarely within the medical model. This is because the medical or "disease" model assumes that violent behavior is associated with an abnormality in neurological or biochemical function. What are the implications of treating violent behavior as a disease or abnormality within the individual, as opposed to looking for social causes and possible corrections?

In the present context, we need to know what constitutes expertise in the area of violence. Who are the experts on violence (psychiatrists? criminologists? social scientists?), and what should their role be in decisions that affect the public regarding research programs? More generally, who should make policy decisions governing research on antisocial and violent behavior? Two factors need to be considered in this connection. First, there is the nature of research subjects and the fact that their participation is not always fully voluntary. How are the rights of research subjects—for the most part, prisoners and mental patients—to be protected? Second, the source of funding for research: When tax dollars are used for research efforts in questionable or volatile areas, it is frequently argued that public participation of some sort in policy decisions is morally necessary as well as politically expedient.

Once it is decided that some community involvement is desirable or even morally required, it becomes necessary to determine the most appropriate spokesmen for the community or for the public at large. The broadest question about expertise and public participation in policy decisions concerning research on violence is this: What ought to be the relationship between researchers, their subjects, and the community?

The UCLA Episode

All these general themes and policy issues played a role in the activities preventing the opening of the UCLA Center for the Study and Reduction of Violence. The main features were as follows.[6] Beginning in September 1972, a series of proposals for research on violent behavior were prepared by faculty members of the Neuropsychiatric Institute at UCLA. An early document proposed to study experimental subjects "in the community, in prisons, in mental hospitals, or wherever practicable." The proposed areas of research included genetic, biochemical, neurological, and neurophysiological investigations. This same document referred to the procedure of electrode implantation as an object of study, claiming that:

> it is even possible to record bioelectrical changes in the brains of freely moving subjects, through the use of remote monitoring techniques. These methods . . . are not yet feasible for large-scale screening that might permit detection of violence-predisposing brain disorders prior to the occurrence of a violent episode. A major task of the Center should be to devise such a test, perhaps sharpened in its predictive powers by correlated measures of psychological test results, biochemical changes in urine or blood, etc. (p. 2)

Publicity for the proposed research center began early in 1973. An article in the *San Francisco Chronicle* mentioned that prison inmates might be used as volunteer subjects in the Center. According to Louis J. West, Director of the Neuropsychiatric Institute, "that was when the trouble began." Among the opponents of the proposed Center beginning to emerge at this time were spokesmen for the Committee Opposing Psychiatric Abuse of Prisoners (COPAP).

Some time later, Dr. West communicated with the Director of Health for the State of California, informing him of the availability of an abandoned Nike missile base located in the Santa Monica mountains, within a half-hour's drive of the Neuropsychiatric Institute. West claimed that this site could be put to very good use as a research facility because of its accessibility and relative remoteness. The site was securely fenced and suitable for prompt occupancy. Among the experimental or model programs for the alteration of undesirable behavior that West suggested might be carried out there were control of drug or alcohol abuse and modification of chronic antisocial or impulsive aggressiveness. West also reported that the Nike base could be used for conferences or retreats for instruction of selected groups of mental health–related professionals, law enforcement personnel, parole officers, and special educators.

By this time, activist groups in addition to COPAP were expressing opposi-

---

[6]The following material describing the UCLA episode and quotations by the principals are taken from unpublished research documents prepared for a conference held at The Hastings Center in February, 1978. Tabitha M. Powledge did the research and wrote the reports as parts of a project entitled "The Dynamics of Scientific Research: Three Case Studies of Scientific Research on Aggression," conducted by the Behavioral Studies Research Group. The project was supported by a grant from the EVIST Program of the National Science Foundation, grant 0SS77–17072. This study was part of the same project that explored the behavior modification programs in prisons described in Chapter 5.

tion to the proposed Center. Members of Students for a Democratic Society distributed leaflets on campus and further events were reported in the UCLA student newspaper. A couple of months later, opposition developed in the California State Assembly, based on the perceived lack of safeguards for human research subjects at the proposed Center. In May 1973, the American Civil Liberties Union expressed concern over the Center, posing the query: "who [sic] does our society view as violent?"

During the same month, this volatile issue came to the attention of members of the American Psychiatric Association through a handout signed by several psychiatrists and distributed at the Association's meeting in Honolulu. The flyer claimed that "the main problem with such a Center is that violence as a social phenomenon, even if lip service is paid to this concept, is pushed to backstage, while the biology or psychology of certain individuals is limelighted." In addition, it claimed, "The proposed Center poses the danger that psychiatrists will be maneuvered increasingly into the position of being used as agents of social control." It is significant that psychiatrists themselves questioned the use of the medical model in this connection and feared the encroachment of their profession into the domain of social control.

The political character of opposition to the Center was evidenced by the fact that the State Senate Health and Welfare Committee held a hearing on the Violence Center. Among those testifying was an attorney who represented the NAACP, the Black Panthers, the National Organization for Women, the Mexican-American Political Association, and the California Prisoners Union. A short time later, the President of the American Civil Liberties Union of Southern California recommended that, on civil liberties grounds, the proposal for establishing the Violence Center should not be funded. Additional political opposition was voiced by the American Friends Service Committee and the Federation of American Scientists.

Since part of the funding for the Center was to come from the Law Enforcement Assistance Administration, an arm of the United States Department of Justice, political involvement soon reached the federal level. Senator Sam Ervin had made an initial inquiry about the Center, and there followed an exchange of letters between Senator Ervin and administrators of the LEAA. Ervin noted in a letter written in January that "programs are being contemplated for the Center that raise profound moral and constitutional questions. . . ." The letters also stated that "there is a serious issue of whether the federal government should be in the position of financing programs posing such extraordinary challenges to human freedom and dignity at all."

The Center for the Study and Reduction of Violence at UCLA never opened. The opposition forces, while never forming a coalition, nonetheless had sufficient political impact to block funding for this project. There were fears expressed on moral grounds about invasive procedures like psychosurgery, electrode implantation, and modes of aversive conditioning. In addition, political opposition arose out of the concerns of special groups such as prisoners, minorities, and dissident students. The establishment of this Center thus became a political football as well as a moral issue. A great many psychiatrists were involved in one way or another in the events surrounding the attempt to set up this research facility. Moreover, they were lined up on both sides of the fence: against as well as for the Center. Plans to seek further funding for the Center as originally proposed were dropped, in the face of continuing opposition and gloomy prospects for financial support. But Dr. West and his colleagues at the Neuropsychiatric Institute have gone forward with at least some of the projects described in the various proposals for the Center, and have sought funds from other federal agencies to carry out research originally planned under the auspices of the proposed Center.

The CIA and Mind Control

The controversy surrounding the UCLA Center for the Study and Reduction of Violence raises moral and political questions about the proper role of psychiatry. Research and development techniques for predicting and controlling violent behavior have as their primary application some form of social control. As we saw earlier, psychiatrists who work in institutions inevitably face double-agent problems when they adhere to accepted diagnostic and treatment practices. But the behavior-control stories that stunned public officials and private citizens the most, when the press began to unfold the tale, were the collaborative efforts between psychiatrists, psychologists, and the Central Intelligence Agency.[7]

Both similarities and differences exist between research and treatment carried out by mental health workers in a typical institutional setting and activities where they are paid agents in secret government operations. Problems of conflicting loyalty arise in both contexts. Balancing the importance of a particular piece of research against the risk of harm to human subjects is another similarity. But the differences far outweigh the similarities. Recent reports of behavior-control research sponsored by the CIA over a period of several decades reveal wide-ranging investigations on prisoners, mental patients, military personnel, and others. Many of these studies were carried out on unwitting subjects, with no attempt to gain their informed consent. In addition, experiments conducted on some of these subjects resulted in their death or permanent mental disability. Research of this sort is considered unethical by the professions themselves, and would probably be unacceptable according to the rules of the American Psychiatric Association and the American Psychological Association, as well as being in violation of current federal regulations governing research on human subjects.

The point here is not, however, to recount another saga of horror stories about human experimentation. It is, rather, to analyze the actions of psychiatrists and psychologists engaged in secret behavior control research under CIA auspices. Does loyalty to one's country justify mounting research efforts that could make cooperating mental health professionals agents of unprecedented social control? The tale of psychiatrists who collaborated with the CIA on a variety of experiments is as much a story of double agency as it is a case of eager researchers with unbounded curiosity who saw a chance to embark with impunity on mind-control projects of an exotic nature.

Reporters from *The New York Times* and independent investigators in the late 1970s uncovered new information about CIA research on behavior and thought control. Even before these latest findings, the agency's work in this area was known to some extent. The newly discovered information included the cost of the program,

---

[7]The following material describing the CIA research on "mind control" was taken from articles in *The New York Times* dated August 2, 1977, and can be found in a recently published book by John Marks, entitled *The Search for the "Manchurian Candidate"* (Times Books, a division of Quadrangle), The New York Times Book Co., Inc., 1979.

the involvement of several prestigious research centers, a number of secret funding conduits, and suppression of deep concerns expressed by some scientists about a number of research programs. In addition, it was learned that the CIA paid for studies conducted by other government agencies and had connections, as well, with behavior control experiments carried out by the armed forces.

In some instances participating psychiatrists, psychologists, and other researchers knew of the sources of funds and the CIA involvement. In other cases they were unaware that the funding sources for their investigations were linked to the CIA. One biopsychiatrist, known for his research on the pleasure center of the brain, was approached by a CIA doctor in 1962 and asked whether he would be interested in exploring the "pain center" of the brain. The psychiatrist, chairman of the Tulane University department of psychiatry and neurology, refused the request, calling it "abhorrent." In his own research, this psychiatrist had performed psychosurgery and had done work on implanting electrodes into the brain. Those investigations were part of a research program seeking ways to treat schizophrenic patients. Yet when approached by the chief of the CIA's medical service division, who said that the Russians were investigating the pain center of the brain and that funds could be provided for this sort of medical research, the psychiatrist stated: "If I were going to be a spy, I'd be a spy. I wanted to be a doctor and practice medicine." He said he felt such work violated the physicians' Hippocratic Oath because it promised no benefit to the patient or mankind.

It is worth noting that it was not the medical procedures themselves to which this psychiatrist objected when approached by the CIA doctor. He was already engaged in research on psychosurgery and on ESB—research directed at locating and understanding more about the pleasure and pain centers of the brain. But this physician saw the aim of his work to be therapy. The CIA request was unambiguously designed for social control and was therefore unacceptable to a doctor who saw his proper role as serving in a therapeutic capacity.

Other medical researchers expressed similar reactions upon learning that a research corporation set up to fund a study of brainwashing was connected with the CIA. Several psychiatric investigators from Cornell University Medical School pulled out of the research corporation, with one of them claiming that funds were "being used in ways that didn't seem consonant with the role of a medical center." Another researcher described brainwashing experiments conducted on patients at the Allan Memorial Institute of Psychiatry at McGill University in Montreal. He recounted experiments done on nonpatients as well, one of which was a sensory-deprivation study conducted on nurses. One nurse suffered a severe reaction, thinking snakes were coming out from under her chair. Months later she was diagnosed as schizophrenic and hospitalized. This researcher, too, claimed to have no knowledge of the CIA connection.

But although many researchers appeared to have no knowledge that their work was funded by the CIA or that their results were intended for nonmedical purposes, an equal number were aware of the Central Intelligence Agency role. Dr. Louis J. West, whose role in the UCLA Violence Center was described earlier, was asked by an employee of the CIA to make a study of LSD. West was aware of the CIA involvement and said he felt they had a legitimate interest in the problem at that time. Another physician, described by the *Times* as "an eager experimenter," also did research on LSD and other drugs that the agency wanted tested. In secret correspondence with his CIA contact, this researcher stated: "I will write you a quick letter as soon as I can get the stuff into a man or two." This research on mind-altering drugs was carried out between 1952 and 1963 on prisoners at the United States Public Health Service hospital in Lexington, Kentucky.

Other LSD experiments for the CIA were conducted on prisoners at the Federal penitentiary in Atlanta and at the Bordentown Reformatory in New Jersey between 1955 and 1964. Experiments using tranquilizers and alcohol on mental patients and staff members of the Butler Memorial Hospital in Providence, Rhode Island, were done on behalf of the CIA. One researcher, knowing of the CIA connection, maintained that the LSD research he conducted on 80 to 100 prisoners at the Atlanta prison and the Bordentown reformatory was done with fully informed consent of the subjects. He added, though, that administering LSD to unwitting subjects might be justified under wartime conditions.

Some of this research sponsored by the CIA, known under the code name "Project Bluebird/Artichoke," was conducted through private medical research foundations. Some was done through the military. According to some reports, subjects granted full and informed consent for the experiments. In most cases, those subjected to mind-altering drugs, sensory-deprivation studies, and brainwashing experiments had no knowledge either that they were serving as experimental subjects or what the research was for. Some studies were done on prisoners, mental patients, and other captive populations. Other tests were conducted on military personnel and staff members at psychiatric hospitals and research centers. In one instance, inmates termed "sexual psychopaths" at the Iona State Hospital in Michigan were given LSD and a marijuana derivative in an attempt to uncover their most secret thoughts. Available evidence indicates that neither the CIA nor the researchers obtained informed consent from these experimental subjects. What is striking about this episode is that the subjects were selected from the files of the Detroit Recorder's Court Psychiatric Clinic. It appears that state judges were informed about the intelligence agency's interest in the tests. In sum, the CIA was engaged in a morally suspect 25-year, $25-million effort to learn how to control the human mind.

Hindsight reveals that the agency never found "the secret of mind control." Documents recently made public demonstrate that it had little success with interrogation using drugs and hypnosis. But it would be a mistake to conclude that these experiments might have been warranted had they resulted in scientifically valuable information. Even among CIA officials, concern was voiced about the ethics and the legality of their contemplated experiments. The Nuremberg Code of Medical Ethics, which emerged from the Nuremberg trials for Nazi war criminals, was adopted by the United States government in 1953. By the early 1960s, the CIA had grown uncomfortable about the experiments. Yet they continued at least through the late 1960s, if not into the 1970s.

More difficult to justify than the CIA's role in research on mind control is the activity of those psychiatrists and other investigators who proceeded with full knowledge of the source of funding and the uses to which experimental results would be put. Even apart from the ethical issue raised by failure to obtain informed consent, these behavior-control researchers were not employees of the CIA, the military, or the federal government. They were not, therefore, placed in the classic double-agent position. Were there imminent threat of aggression or violence—from within or without—an argument could be offered in support of such research efforts. Based on the need to preserve the very existence of our society, or at least our present way of life, such an argument might initially seem plausible. But to show even this much, the argument would have to account for at least the following elements. There would have to be good evidence that an imminent threat existed; that this behavior-control research would be likely to thwart efforts mounted by foreign powers; that no alternative measures would be at least as successful against the impending threats; and that the violation of the rights of human subjects and the risks of harm through experimentation would be outweighed by the benefits of the research.

Given these requirements, it seems unlikely that facts and probabilities could be marshalled in support of an argument justifying the CIA's research projects on behavior control. The empirical evidence required to draw such a conclusion on utilitarian grounds is surely lacking. The presumed need for such research stems from the threat to our way of life posed by invasions from hostile powers. The CIA's rationale for the research it promoted was that the Russians were doing it. In the early 1950s, "brainwashing" techniques and "thought reform" practiced on American soldiers captured during the Korean conflict were viewed with alarm. But if the way of life we want so much to preserve permits the type of experiments devised by the CIA, conducted on vulnerable populations of mostly unwitting subjects, with the cooperation of respected psychiatrists and other researchers in behavior control, we had best rethink what it is we cherish so much in our way of life.

Policy Decisions in Behavior Control

Both research and treatment in the domain of behavior control require careful monitoring in a free society. The UCLA experience shows that even the best-intentioned psychiatrists may fail to appreciate how their efforts to study and control violence will be perceived by special-interest groups, the public at large, and other psychiatrists. Research activities of the CIA demonstrate that some psychiatrists may become unknowing dupes of zealous government agents, while others are prepared to cooperate in morally questionable practices. Many behavior-control experts firmly believe that the causes of violence lie within the brain, and direct their research and therapeutic practices accordingly. It needs no reminder that the authority of the psychiatric profession generally affords its members with the power to make decisions that profoundly affect the lives of hospitalized mental patients, prisoners, suicidal persons, and completely free individuals judged dangerous to others.

It may seem paradoxical to suggest that in a free society those authorized to conduct research and treatment for controlling human behavior ought to be subjected to some form of control themselves. The freedom to pursue research in an unfettered manner has been a hallmark of scientific practice in our society. Recent concern over the protection of human subjects of biomedical and behavioral research has led to new regulations and stricter enforcement of old ones—a development not universally welcomed by physicians and scientists who feel themselves under greater constraints than before. Freedom to seek new knowledge should be protected too, these scientists urge, since the results of research stand to affect society in positive ways. Many investigators feel strongly that the pendulum has swung too far—that freedom of scientific inquiry has been hampered.

After much attention to the question of whether certain types of research ought to be allowed to go forward, the reverse question is now being raised in many quarters: What are the consequences of halting research that may prove beneficial?

This query has been directed at experimental behavior-modification programs in prisons; at the studies planned for the UCLA Violence Center; and at a variety of research efforts on prisoners designed to investigate the way hormones contribute to the tendency to commit or refrain from committing sexual assaults. It is even possible that some thinking persons lamented the cessation of the CIA research efforts to control the mind.

What are the consequences of halting research aimed at controlling or altering human behavior? The answer depends primarily on two factors: first, the likelihood that the research will prove fruitful; and second, the risks of harm that may result from engaging in the research. This second factor breaks down into two further parts: the possibility of harm resulting from the research itself, as in the suicide of an unwitting subject of the CIA experiments with LSD; and longer term consequences, such as a breakdown in trust of psychiatrists and others who propose or engage in research projects.

Risks and Benefits of Research

The need to make assessments of risks and gains poses many difficulties. In the first place, if research is breaking ground—if it is truly frontier research—surely its fruitfulness cannot be demonstrated in advance. But in the absence of advance knowledge of whether a particular piece of research will prove fruitful, how can we answer the question "what are the consequences of halting research?" As for the second factor—the risks of harm to research subjects or other untoward consequences that may result—this is the point of so-called risk-benefit equations that human investigations committees are charged with assessing. The need to weigh probable benefits of research against probable risks may look like an exercise in first-year algebra: Fill in the risk-benefit variables in the equation and solve for x. Yet it is precisely the difficulty of performing this balancing act that leads to one of the conflicts over research on the causes and control of violent behavior.

What are the losses that could result from halting research on the causes and control of violent behavior? One possible loss might be the failure to develop ethically and socially satisfactory alternatives to incarceration. When the Neuropsychiatric Institute at UCLA submitted its first official grant proposal in April 1973, it included a section on Determinants of Violence as one of the research and development aspects of the proposed studies. As specified in the proposal, the task was

> ... to develop models for the prediction of the probability of subsequent violence in individuals concerning whom a decision must be made whether to hold the individual in a situation where relatively extensive external controls exist, or to utilize minimal external controls, or to release the individuals with minimal external controls.

The emphasis here is on research that could lead to more accurate predictions of violent behavior.

Yet even if it would be a real gain if research on violence led to a greater degree of predictability, questions still remain about the uses to which such knowledge would be put. Advances in scientific knowledge are usually thought of as benefits. But it is well known that morally neutral knowledge may be applied in ways that are at least morally questionable, if not clearly unethical.

Inevitably, we are led back to the question: Can the potential benefits and dangers of high-risk research be anticipated? As with so many other queries posed throughout this book, the answer is: Sometimes yes, sometimes no. Part of the uncertainty lies in the fact that considerable disagreement persists over what is to count as a benefit. Few would disagree with the proposition that it would be a good thing if less violence were committed against innocent persons in our society. But if we dig a layer deeper and examine specific forms of research on violence, who is likely to engage in such research, and what its applications might be, then disagreement begins to mount over what should count as a benefit and what could properly be thought of as harm stemming from behavior control research. Often, it is a case of weighing one harm against another.

Research on violence and aggression is considered by many to be potentially dangerous research. The dangers may lie in the actual conduct of the research, as was the case with subjects harmed in the course of the CIA studies on the effects of LSD and of sensory deprivation. Or it may lie in abuses that occur later as a result of applying knowledge gained from research, such as the use of succinylcholine as an aversive stimulus in coercive treatment programs in prisons designed to modify the behavior of criminal offenders. Another type of danger is the sort that may stem from political outcries and power plays by groups who feel threatened, as occurred in the flare-up over the UCLA Violence Center.

Empirical, ethical, and conceptual uncertainty often makes it hard to tell in advance when a particular research effort is subject to abuse. In the first chapter, we observed that the number of competing theories in psychology and psychiatry is legion. No well-confirmed, generally agreed-upon theory of human behavior exists today. In the absence of a strong theoretical basis for continued research on violence and aggression, it is no wonder that unanswered questions and ill-formulated objections abound. Bearing in mind the state of ignorance about the causes of violence reported by "expert" witnesses before the House of Representatives subcommittee, we can more easily understand the controversies that arise over potential abuses of behavior control research.

A familiar point from the philosophy of science deserves mention here: Empirical data do not uniquely determine a specific theory. Consistent data derived from research may be compatible with a variety of scientific theories invoked to explain the data. In more advanced stages of scientific inquiry, a complete, systematic theory serves to structure and organize the empirical data. But in the study of human behavior—a field still in its infancy—there is bound to be uncertainty and disagreement over both theory and applications of research data. Until these theoretical and empirical gaps in knowledge are closed, it is impossible to make conclusive judgments about the ethics of research on violent behavior—its causes and control.

Lessons for the Future

What, then, should we conclude about embattled research and controversial treatment programs? Should they continue to go forward in the future, regardless of the likelihood of conflicts and disagreements like those that emerged in the past? Or is it better to cease such efforts in the belief that they are bound to become politicized and to arouse moral objections?

The ultimate practical decisions in this domain depend on what sort of life we as a society want to pursue. Is the best society one that is willing to undergo some risks of harm to individuals or to restrict some personal freedoms in the hopes of potential long-range benefits? Or does scientific progress in the control of human behavior become a questionable goal if it can only be won at the expense of invading the privacy, autonomy, and dignity of some of society's members? In a free and democratic society, the political process ultimately resolves these moral issues. Ideally, a knowledgeable and enlightened public is more likely to reach rational and reflective conclusions about policy matters in any area than a society kept in the dark about scientific research and its applications. Control of human behavior is an especially sensitive area, and so a public ignorant of the relevant facts is likely to react out of blind prejudice or blatant misconceptions.

Any procedure or technological advance may be subject to abuse or misuse, but that fact alone is usually not sufficient to justify banning such practices altogether. Since research and applications in behavior control so readily become hot political issues, the question "who should decide?" remains in the forefront. The general presumption in a democracy lies with the public. Where individual decisions require psychiatric or psychological expertise—such as the best way of treating a chronically depressed person or one who suffers severe anxiety—there should be little doubt about the appropriateness of decision making by qualified mental health professionals. But when psychiatrists abandon their primary role as healers and become, instead, agents of social control—then there is serious room for doubt about their expertise for making decisions that set behavior control policies.

People become wary when scientific and social issues get politicized. But is that development always a bad thing? It is the mark of a pluralistic society that different interest groups seek power and insist on receiving their due. It is a characteristic of democracy that the "will of the people" should prevail. In the realm of behavior control, the public appears to have numerous and divergent wills. It seems most appropriate in a free society for issues that raise ethical, social, and political concerns to be settled by the democratic process. If we want to hold on to the freedom and democracy that have served as ideals in our society, even if they are not always fully practiced, we cannot afford to leave policy decisions about behavior control solely in the hands of behavior-control experts. In many areas, the ways of the brain and behavior remain mysteries. Future gains will not be limited to scientific advances in understanding, prediction, and control. Hopes for the future also lie in bringing to an informed public the concerns that affect us all. Ethical decisions are not best accomplished by majority rule, any more than by the exercise of society's elite members. We need free, open, and informed discussion, so that our society can evolve moral principles appropriate to new theoretical and technological advances in the sphere of behavior control.

FURTHER READINGS

NATIONAL COMMISSION FOR THE PROTECTION OF HUMAN SUBJECTS, *Psychosurgery: Report and Recommendations* and *Appendix*. Washington, D.C.: U.S. Department of Health, Education, and Welfare, 1977.

———, *Research Involving Prisoners: Report and Recommendations* and *Appendix*. Washington, D.C.: U.S. Department of Health, Education, and Welfare, 1976.

———, *Research Involving Those Institutionalized as Mentally Infirm: Report and Recommendations* and *Appendix*. Washington, D.C.: U.S. Department of Health, Education, and Welfare, 1976.

Index